The Tibial Plateu Fractures: Diagnosis and Treatment

Francesco Atzori

University of Turin, Unit of Orthopaedics and Traumatology
Hospital San Luigi Gonzaga
Regione Gonzole 10, 10043, Orbassano (Turin)
Italy

Luigi Sabatini

University of Turin, Unit of Orthopaedics and Traumatology
Hospital San Luigi Gonzaga
Regione Gonzole 10, 10043, Orbassano (Turin)
Italy

advertisements or ideas contained in the Work.

Limitation of Liability:

In no event will Bentham Science Publishers, its staff, editors and/or authors, be liable for any damages, including, without limitation, special, incidental and/or consequential damages and/or damages for lost data and/or profits arising out of (whether directly or indirectly) the use or inability to use the Work. The entire liability of Bentham Science Publishers shall be limited to the amount actually paid by you for the Work.

General:

1. Any dispute or claim arising out of or in connection with this License Agreement or the Work (including non-contractual disputes or claims) will be governed by and construed in accordance with the laws of the U.A.E. as applied in the Emirate of Dubai. Each party agrees that the courts of the Emirate of Dubai shall have exclusive jurisdiction to settle any dispute or claim arising out of or in connection with this License Agreement or the Work (including non-contractual disputes or claims).

2. Your rights under this License Agreement will automatically terminate without notice and without the need for a court order if at any point you breach any terms of this License Agreement. In no event will any delay or failure by Bentham Science Publishers in enforcing your compliance with this License Agreement constitute a waiver of any of its rights.

3. You acknowledge that you have read this License Agreement, and agree to be bound by its terms and conditions. To the extent that any other terms and conditions presented on any website of Bentham Science Publishers conflict with, or are inconsistent with, the terms and conditions set out in this License Agreement, you acknowledge that the terms and conditions set out in this License Agreement shall prevail.

Bentham Science Publishers Ltd.
Executive Suite Y - 2
PO Box 7917, Saif Zone
Sharjah, U.A.E.
Email: subscriptions@benthamscience.org

BENTHAM SCIENCE

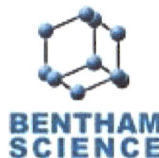

CONTENTS

DEDICATION

Dedicated to whom we love and to those who love us.

PREFACE

The importance of this argument arises from high incidence of tibial plateau fractures, from epidemiology of this kind of fracture (usually young and active people) and from necessity to obtain a good restoration of function.

Tibial plateau fractures are mostly articular fractures. The goal of treatment is restoration of function and fracture fixation must offer enough stability to allow early mobilisation.

Several problems are correlated to this kind of fracture:

- cutaneous and soft tissue damage are often present, as these fractures often result from high energy trauma
- diagnosis is sometimes difficult: x-ray, CT scans and MRI can be used without a correct standardization
- associated lesions of menisci or ligaments can influence the final outcome
- different procedures are described for tibial plateau fractures: conservative treatment, open reduction and internal fixation, with arthroscopic techniques, with external fixation, using "balloon" indirect reduction, *etc.*
- postoperative care is fundamental to obtain a good result, but the timing is not so clear

We think a book clarifying and summarizing anatomy, pathogenesis, diagnosis, treatment and rehabilitation can help all orthopaedics surgeons treating this disabling kind of fracture. Our objective is not to give a definitive answer about treatment choice, but to propose some solutions on the basis of the fracture "personality".

Francesco Atzori
University of Turin
Italy

&

Luigi Sabatini
University of Turin
Italy

FOREWORD

It is a great pleasure to write the foreword for *"The tibial plateu fractures: diagnosis and treatment"*, edited by my colleagues and friends Francesco Atzori and Luigi Sabatini.

Techniques in traumatic knee surgery have continued to evolve and the editors of this book have described various possible surgical procedures. The authors articulate with clarity the best evidence available to support the use of the procedure they described as well as any controversial aspects of the technique and alternative treatment options if available.

Furthermore, every perspective of tibial plateau fractures is well represented, from epidemiology to rehabilitation protocols.

I think this e-book will be extremely precious for every orthopaedic surgeon, residents and fellows to manage tibial plateau fractures and I congratulate the Editors and the Authors on the production of a very interesting e-book.

Marco Schiraldi
Unit Orthopaedics and Traumatology
Orthopaedic Prostethic Surgery Regional Center
Hospital SS. Antonio e Biagio e Cesare Arrigo
Alessandria
Italy
Email: mschiraldi@ospedale.al.it

List of Contributors

Angelino Valeria	University of Turin, Radiology Department, Hospital San Luigi Gonzaga, Regione Gonzole 10, 10043, Orbassano (Turin), Italy
Aprato Alessandro	University of Turin, Unit of Orthopaedics and Traumatology, Hospital San Luigi Gonzaga, Regione Gonzole 10, 10043, Orbassano (Turin), Italy
Atzori Francesco	University of Turin, Unit of Orthopaedics and Traumatology, Hospital San Luigi Gonzaga, Regione Gonzole 10, 10043, Orbassano (Turin), Italy
Azi Matheus	Manoel Victorino Hospital, Pc Conselheiro Almeida Couto, s/n Largo de Nazaré, Nazaré , Salvador, Brasil
Barbin Robert	Gold Coast University Hospital, 1 Hospital Boulevard, Southport, Australia
Bistolfi Alessandro	University of Turin, Department of Orthopaedic and Traumatology, C.T.O. Hospital, *Via* Gianfranco Zuretti 29, 10126 Turin, Italy
Bruzzone Matteo	University of Turin, Department of Orthopaedic and Traumatology, Hospital Mauriziano Umberto I, Largo Turati 62, 10128 Torino (TO), Italy
Busso Marco	University of Turin, Radiology Department, Hospital San Luigi Gonzaga, Regione Gonzole 10, 10043 Orbassano, Turin, Italy
Carnino Irene	School of Rehabilitative Medicine, University of the Studies of Turin, *Via* Po 8, 10100 Turin , Italy
Colonese Francesca	University of Turin, Radiology Department, Hospital San Luigi Gonzaga, Regione Gonzole 10, 10043 Orbassano, Turin, Italy
Cottino Umberto	School of Orthopaedics and Traumatology, University of Turin, *Via* Po 8, 10100 Turin, Italy
Deledda Davide	School of Orthopaedics and Traumatology, University of Turin, *Via* Po 8, 10100 Turin, Italy
Dettoni Federico	University of Turin, Department of Orthopaedic and Traumatology, Hospital Mauriziano Umberto I, Largo Turati 62, 10128 Torino, Italy
Dolfin Marco	Unit of Orthopaedics and Traumatology, Hospital San Giovanni Bosco, Piazza Del Donatore Del Sangue 3, 10154 Turin, Italy
Martino Deregibus	School of Orthopaedics and Traumatology, University of Turin, *Via* Po 8, 10100 Turin , Italy
Federico Annamaria	School of Rehabilitative Medicine, University of the Studies of Turin, *Via* Po 8, 10100 Turin, Italy
Gaido Cecilia	School of Rehabilitative Medicine, University of the Studies of Turin, *Via* Po 8, 10100 Turin, Italy

Giachino Matteo	School of Orthopaedics and Traumatology, University of Turin, *Via* Po 8, 10100 Turin, Italy
Jayasekara Narlaka	Department of Orthopaedics, Gold Coast University Hospital, 1 Hospital Boulevard, Southport, Australia
Massazza Giuseppe	University of Turin, Department of Orthopaedic and Traumatology, C.T.O. Hospital, *Via* Gianfranco Zuretti 29, 10126 Turin , Italy
Massè Alessandro	University of Turin, Director of Unit of Orthopaedics and Traumatology, Hospital San Luigi Gonzaga - Regione Gonzole 10, 10043 Orbassano, Turin, Italy
Rossi Roberto	University of Turin, Department of Orthopaedic and Traumatology Director, Hospital Mauriziano Umberto I, Largo Turati 62, 10128 Torino , Italy
Rosso Federica	School of Orthopaedics and Traumatology, University of Turin, *Via* Po 8, 10100 Turin , Italy
Sabatini Luigi	University of Turin, Unit of Orthopaedics and Traumatology, Hospital San Luigi Gonzaga, Regione Gonzole 10, 10043 Orbassano, Italy
Saccia Francesco	Unit of Orthopaedics and Traumatology, Hospital San Giovanni Bosco, Piazza Del Donatore Del Sangue 3, 10154 Turin, Italy
Salama Wael	Orthopaedic Department, Sohag University Hospital (SUH), Sohag 82524, Egypt
Santoro Daniele	University of Turin, Unit of Traumatology, C.T.O. Hospital - *Via* Gianfranco Zuretti 29, 10126 Turin , Italy
Singh Jaswinder	Unit of Orthopaedics and Traumatology, Medical College, Brown Road, Ludhiana, India
Torre Federico	University of Turin, Radiology Department, Hospital San Luigi Gonzaga - Regione Gonzole 10, 10043 Orbassano , Italy
Trikha Vivek	Department of Orthopaedics, All India Institute of Medical Sciences, New Delhi 110029, India
Veltri Andrea	University of Turin, Director of Radiology Department Unit, Hospital San Luigi Gonzaga, Regione Gonzole 10, 10043 Orbassano, Italy
Vijayan Sridhar	Gold Coast University Hospital, 1 Hospital Boulevard , Southport, Australia

The Tibial Plateu Fractures: Diagnosis and Treatment

2

TheTibial Plateu Fractures :Diagnosis and Treatment

Editors: Francesco Atzori, Luigi Sabatini

ISBN (eBook): 978-1-68108-241-7

ISBN (Print): 978-1-68108-242-4 © 2016, Bentham eBooks imprint.

Published by Bentham Science Publishers – Sharjah, UAE. All Rights Reserved.

First published in 2016.

CHAPTER 1

Pathogenesis and Epidemiology of Tibial Plateau Fractures

Alessandro Massè[1,*] and **Martino Deregibus[2]**

[1] University of Turin, Unit of Orthopaedics and Traumatology, Hospital San Luigi Gonzaga, Orbassano (Turin), Italy

[2] Unit of Orthopaedics and Traumatology, Hospital Regina Montis Regalis, Mondovì, (Cuneo), Italy

Abstract: Fracture of the tibial plateau is seen frequently in orthopedic trauma units and pose major threats to the structure and function of the knee joint. Tibial plateau fractures are complex injuries to treat due to their articular involvement and associated disruption of ligamentous structures in the knee. For many years several discussion has been done about the best treatment of tibial plateau fractures . A lot of orthopeadic surgeons and researchers have analyzed functional and radiologic results for nonoperative and surgical, treatments [1, 2]. Nevertheless the surgical treatment is mandatory in the tibial platueau fracture associated with an acute compartment syndrome or an acute vascular lesion and in open tibial plateau fracture.

Keywords: Articular fracture, Compartment syndrome, Epidemiology, Mechanism injury, Plateau fracture.

INTRODUCTION

- Tibial plateau is formed by medial and lateral tibial plateaus. They are the articular surfaces of the medial and lateral tibial condyles and they articulate with the medial and lateral femoral condyles, respectively. They are an essential part of knee joint, a diarthrodial joints, which provide a smooth, stable capacity

---

[*] **Correspondence author Alessandro Massè:** University of Turin, Director of Unit of Orthopaedics and Traumatology, Hospital San Luigi Gonzaga, Regione Gonzole 10, 10043, Orbassano (Turin), Italy; Tel: +39.011.9026619; E-mail: alessandro.masse@unito.it

Francesco Atzori and Luigi Sabatini (Eds)

for motion of the appendicular skeleton to perform specialized tasks [3].

- So it is essential to know the general bases for an effective treatment of any articular fracture:

The alteration of the articular surface joint often affect stability, cause pain, and disrupt effective range of motion of the joint. The inflammatory response combined with this type of fracture can create a massive fibrosis within the injured joint, exacerbated by inadequate immobilization or inappropriate surgical treatmentss. The malconsolidation of the fracture was often associated with a bony deformity, stiffness, pain, and functional disability. The anatomical restoration of the articular surface and freedom of joint movement is necessary to obtaine a favorable outcome [3].

EPIDEMIOLOGY

Epidemiology of Tibial Plateau Fracture

The prevalence of tibial plateau fractures is 1.3% of all fractures, males are more often affected than females. Several studies show that 71% of injuries occurred in those aged 30-60 years.

It isn't the most common tibial fracture, having a frequency of less than 10% [4, 5].

Both high energy trauma (*e.g.* motor vehicle, cycling and winter sports) and low energy trauma (*e.g.* falls, contact sports, distance running, and other endurance or repetitive impact activities) are commone causes of this kind of fracture.

It occurs principally in two groups of patient:

Younger or middle-aged patients, suffered of moderate or high-energy injuries (especially motor vehicle accidents or a fall from a height) and elderly osteoporotic patients, who suffered of low energy injury like a simple fall [5, 6].

When tibial plateau fractures are cause by falls from height, they can be associated with calcaneal fractures and fractures of the thoraco-lumbar spine, nevertheless in the majority of cases the lesion is isolated. It affect rarely the children and young adults prior to epiphyseal plate closure.

The principal causes are:

- Road traffic accidents 52%;
- Falls 17%;
- Sporting or recreational activities in 5% [5, 7].

There is a third group, significantly less numerous compared to the previous, regarding stress fracture. Stress fracture are common in military and athletic trainess during running, as they often develop forces that are several times higher than their body weight at the interface between foot and terrain.

Military and athletic trainees population are more mainly affected by stress fractures. During training exercises they can develop forces much higher than their body weight at the interface between foot and ground during running [8].

Epidemiology of Different Type of Tibial Plateau Fracture

Several studies show that 52-68% were low energy lesions (level ≤ 3) while approximately 32-48% of the lesions were caused by a high energy impact, according to Hohl scales (level 5), Schatzker scale (levels 5 and 6) and AO (levels C1, C2 and C3) [2, 4, 9].

Yang *et al.* observed a particular type of lesion, the fracture of the posterior tibial plateau. Posterior tibial plateau fracture (PTPF) was defined as a fracture with an independent fragment of the posterior column. It is associated especially with high energy lesions (Schatzker levels 5 and 6) with percentages of 51.2 and 76.1%, respectively [10].

Epidemiology of Soft Tissue Lesion Associated

It is now widely accepted that the incidence of soft tissue injuries, such as meniscal tears and ligamentous lesions (ACL, PCL, LCL and MCL), are common, ranging from 47% to 99% [11, 12].

The frequency of soft tissue injury has been found to be in direct correlation with the energy of the initial injury, which often translates to fracture classification.

Gardner *et al.* evaluated 103 patients with tibial plateau fractures, investigating soft-tissue injuries by MRI. They highlighted a complete absence of soft tissues injuries in 1% of patients, while up to 91% showed a meniscal injury [13].

Mustonen *et al.* demonstrated an elevated prevalence (36%) of an unstable meniscal tear [14]. Shepherd *et al.* demonstrated an elevated prevalence of meniscal, ligamentous and other soft-tissue injuries even in minimally displaced fractures [11]. Many authors have discussed about the treatments of these soft-tissue for several years. Actually the gold standard treatment aims to create a stable knee, guaranteeing a rapid recover of knee motion and function and minimizing the risk of secondary osteoarthritis in the long term.

There has yet to be a gold standard for accurately predicting the presence of soft tissue injuries in tibial plateau fractures. However, there have been recent studies that have employed preoperative magnetic resonance imaging (MRI) or operative arthroscopy to evaluate the extent of tissue damage [15 - 17].

Red Flag: The Compartment Syndrome

Compartment syndrome is a terrible complication of tibial fractures. The rate of compartment syndrome is highest in the diaphyseal tibial fracture with a rate of 8%. It is less common in proximal and distal fracture. The rate in proximale fracture is less than 2%. Nevertheless tibial plateau fractures, expecially if the diaphisis is involved, can lead to an acute compartment syndromes because of hemorrhage and edema of the muscular compartments [18].

Chang *et al.* demonstrated that the incidence of compartment syndrome seem to be related to the fracture pattern as well as to the mechanism of trauma. The compartment syndrome was more common in high-energy traumas (Schatzker's type IV, V, and VI), ranging from 30.4% in type VI [19, 20].

Particular Case: The Floating Knee

The floating knee is the ipsilateral fracture of the femur and tibia. It's an uncommon and serious injury which is often associated with other major injuries. The tibial plateau is involved in the type IIa and IIc of floating knee. The rate of these types of lesion is around the 20% of total.

In these cases several studies report an higher rate of complication, an higher rate of open fracture and a worse prognosis than the type I [21, 22].

Most Common Features of Clinical Presentation

- Gender: male,
- Age: fifth decade of life,
- Type of trauma: victim of traffic accidents,
- Type of fracture: depression and shear fractures of the tibial plateau

Mechanism of Injury

General Principle

There are two common mechanisms of injury for articular fractures [3]:

- Direct application of the force
- Indirect application of the force

There is then a third one, less common, that involves especially the athletes [8]:

- Cronic overload

Indirect Application of the Force

Usually the injury is produced by the indirect application of the force, causing a bending moment through the joint. This mechanism bring a part of the joint toward its opposite surface. The ligaments generally resist to the eccentric load, converting the force into a direct axial overload that causes a joint fracture.

Typically, the result is a partial articular fracture [3].

Direct Application of the Force

The other possibile mechanism is the direct application of the force, which can be either caused by a force toward the metaphyseal-diaphyseal component of the joint or through axial transmission of force from one end segment of bone to the opposing surface. Both cases cause the bone explosion with a dissipation of force into the soft tissues. It results in a multifragmentary articular fractures, with associated severe soft-tissue injuries. The fracture pattern is determined by the position of the limb, the bone quality, and the vector of the force applied [3].

Cronic Overload

The third mechanism of injury, significantly less frequent is the repetitive cyclical absorption by bone (tibial bone in this particurarly case) of large compression and tension force developed during walking and running. It thought to produce stress fractures [8, 23].

Mechanism of Injury: The Tibial Plateau Fracture

At the beginning the appellation of these type of fractures was "the fender fracture" because they was principally caused by low-energy pedestrian *versus* car bumper accidents [24, 25].

Injuries to the plateaus occur as a result of:

1. A force directed laterally (varus deformity) or medially (valgus deformity) [see before: indirect application of the force];
2. An axial compressive force [see before: direct application of the force];
3. Both a force from the side and an axial force.

It occurs usually as a consequence of bending and vertical thrust combined. This mechanism of fracture usually causes different combinations of articular surface depressions.

The most common combination of forces is a direct axial compression with a valgus moment and indirect shear forces.

The anterior part of the femoral condyles has got a wedge aspect. When the injury occurs during the knee extension phase, a force that pushes the condyle into the tibial plateau is produced [26]. The fracture pattern is determined by the entity of the phenomenon, in terms of magnitude and location of the force.

The femoral condyles has an anterior wedge shaped aspect. When the knee is in full extension, the force generated by the injury drives the condyle toward the tibial plateau [26]. To determine the fracture pattern is important to understand the direction, magnitude and location of the force. Moreover, the position of the knee during the impact determines the fracture pattern, location, and degree of displacement.

Due to the special anatomic configuration of the knee (valgus position, trabecular pattern of lateral condyle and shape of respective condyle) and the mechanism of injury (the force involved usually is direct from the lateral side to medial part of the knee), up to 55 to 72% of tibial condyle fractures are located laterally [2, 4, 6, 27, 28].

The fracture pattern can also be influenced by patient factors such as age and bone quality.

Depression-type fractures are more frequent in elderly population with osteopenic bone [29] because their subchondral bone is less able to withstand axially directed loads. These are fractures that generally occur after low-energy injuries, as simple slip or fall accidents [30] Younger parients are more likely to sustaina pure split fractures, because they have got a strong subchondral bone of the tibial condyle. It is prone to resist to compressive forces of th overlying femoral condyle, but the shear component of the load can produce a split in the condyle itself [31 - 33].

Biomechanical studies demonstrated how fracture patterns reflect the forces involved.

Kennedy and Bailey [33], using cadaver models, showed many of the commonly observed plateau fracture patterns. They perfomed empirical studies in cadaver knees applying valgus or varus forces in combination with axial loads (ranging from 1600 to 8000 pounds). Mixed fractures with large variations in the amount and degree of joint impaction and condylar separation were generated by valgus loads in the range of 2250 to 3750 inch pounds. These type forces are similar to those seen in the classic tibial plateau fracture (*e.g.* the bumper type). This is a typical fracture of the lateral plateau, that results in a lateral blow to the leg, with a valgus deforming force and a loading of the lateral plateau by the overlying femoral condyle.

After an high-energy injuries, the forces may be so powerful to generate the explosion of the plateau into various fracture fragments. If axial loading exceeded 8000 pounds, the impact produces severely comminuted fractures. This kind of fracture is typically seen after a fall from a height or after a motor vehicle accident, if the axial load is delivered to an extended knee. The magnitude of the force determines the degree of fragmentation and the degree of displacement. Furthermore, an association between tibial plateau fracture and soft tissue lesions is very common:

- A The disruption of anterior cruciate ligament and a tear of medial collateral ligament are associated with a lateral plateu fracture [28, 34].
- The disruption of lateral collateral ligament complex, the posterior cruciate, and the lesion of peroneal nerve or of the popliteal vessels are associated with a medial plateau fracture [34, 35].

Nevertheless, some authors believe that it is necessary an intact collateral ligament on one side of the knee to produce a fracture on the controlateral side [36].

The increase of magnetic resonance imaging (MRI) for these fractures, has improved the recognition of associated ligamentous injuries [11 - 14, 37, 38].

Moreover, it is very important for the surgeon to identify the associated soft tissue lesion and modulate the treatment taking in consideration osseus and soft tissue lesions. It is also crucial to recognize split fractures that are the result of a shearing force from rim avulsion fractures associated with knee dislocations and lead to an unstable injury.

Abstract/Take Home Messages

- Tibial plateau fractures are complex injuries to treat due to their articular involvement and associated disruption of ligamentous structures in the knee.
- It account for 1.3% of all fractures and affect males more commonly than females, it has a frequency of less than 10% of total tibial fractures.
- It occurs in both high energy trauma and low energy trauma.
- The incidence of soft-tissue injuries is high, ranging from 47% to 99%.
- Tibial plateau fractures, especially if they extend into the diaphysis, may be

associated with acute compartment syndromes caused by the hemorrhage and edema of the involved compartments.The rate of compartment syndrome is around 2%.

- Injuries to the plateaus are caused by (1) a force directed either laterally (varus deformity) or medially (valgus deformity, called commonly ''bumper fracture''), (2) an axial compressive force, or (3) both an axial force and a force from the side.

- The complexity of the fracture and the consequent treatment are influenced by the energy transmitted to the limb. Low-energy impact is usually lead to unilateral depression-type fractures, whereas high-energy impact can cause comminuted fractures with important osseous, soft-tissue, and neurovascular injury.

CONFLICT OF INTEREST

The author confirms that author has no conflict of interest to declare for this publication.

ACKNOWLEDGEMENTS

Declared none.

REFERENCES

[1]   Court-Brown CM, McBirnie J. The epidemiology of tibial fractures. J Bone Joint Surg Br 1995; 77(3): 417-21.
        [PMID: 7744927]

[2]   Rademakers MV, Kerkhoffs GM, Sierevelt IN, Raaymakers EL, Marti RK. Operative treatment of 109 tibial plateau fractures: five- to 27-year follow-up results. J Orthop Trauma 2007; 21(1): 5-10.
        [http://dx.doi.org/10.1097/BOT.0b013e31802c5b51] [PMID: 17211262]

[3]   Ruedi TP, Buckley RE, Moran CG. AO principles of fracture management. In: Thomas P, Ruedi TP, Richard E, Buckley RE, Christopher G, Moran CG, Eds. Switzerland: Davos Platz 2007.

[4]   Albuquerque RP, Hara R, Prado J, Schiavo L, Giordano V, do Amaral NP. Epidemiological study on tibial plateau fractures at a level I trauma center. Acta Ortop Bras 2013; 21(2): 109-15.
        [http://dx.doi.org/10.1590/S1413-78522013000200008] [PMID: 24453653]

[5]   Moore TM, Patzakis MJ, Harvey JP. Tibial plateau fractures: definition, demographics, treatment rationale, and long-term results of closed traction management or operative reduction. J Orthop Trauma 1987; 1(2): 97-119.
        [http://dx.doi.org/10.1097/00005131-198702010-00001] [PMID: 3333518]

[6]   Ebraheim NA, Sabry FF, Haman SP. Open reduction and internal fixation of 117 tibial plateau fractures. Orthopedics 2004; 27(12): 1281-7.
        [PMID: 15633959]

[7]   Thomas Ch, Athanasiov A, Wullschleger M, Schuetz M. Current concepts in tibial plateau fractures. Acta Chir Orthop Traumatol Cech 2009; 76(5): 363-73.
        [PMID: 19912699]

[8]   Giladi M, Milgrom C, Simkin A, *et al.* Stress fractures and tibial bone width. A risk factor. J Bone Joint Surg Br 1987; 69(2): 326-9.
        [PMID: 3818769]

[9]   Schatzker J, McBroom R, Bruce D. The tibial plateau fracture. The Toronto experience 1968--1975. Clin Orthop Relat Res 1979; (138): 94-104.
        [PMID: 445923]

[10]   Yang G, Zhai Q, Zhu Y, Sun H, Putnis S, Luo C. The incidence of posterior tibial plateau fracture: an investigation of 525 fractures by using a CT-based classification system. Arch Orthop Trauma Surg 2013; 133(7): 929-34.
        [http://dx.doi.org/10.1007/s00402-013-1735-4] [PMID: 23589062]

[11]   Shepherd L, Abdollahi K, Lee J, Vangsness CT Jr. The prevalence of soft tissue injuries in nonoperative tibial plateau fractures as determined by magnetic resonance imaging. J Orthop Trauma 2002; 16(9): 628-31.
        [http://dx.doi.org/10.1097/00005131-200210000-00003] [PMID: 12368642]

[12]   Zakrzewski P. Or≈Çowski J. Chir Narzadow Ruchu Ortop Pol 2005; 70(2): 109-13. [Meniscuses and ligaments injuries in tibial plateau fractures in comparative evaluation of clinical, intraoperative and MR examination].
        [PMID: 16158867]

[13]   Gardner MJ, Yacoubian S, Geller D, *et al.* The incidence of soft tissue injury in operative tibial plateau fractures: a magnetic resonance imaging analysis of 103 patients. J Orthop Trauma 2005; 19(2): 79-84.
        [http://dx.doi.org/10.1097/00005131-200502000-00002] [PMID: 15677922]

[14]   Mustonen AO, Koivikko MP, Lindahl J, Koskinen SK. MRI of acute meniscal injury associated with tibial plateau fractures: prevalence, type, and location. AJR Am J Roentgenol 2008; 191(4): 1002-9.
        [http://dx.doi.org/10.2214/AJR.07.3811] [PMID: 18806134]

[15]   Stannard JP, Lopez R, Volgas D. Soft tissue injury of the knee after tibial plateau fractures. J Knee Surg 2010; 23(4): 187-92.
        [http://dx.doi.org/10.1055/s-0030-1268694] [PMID: 21446623]

[16]   Markhardt BK, Gross JM, Monu JU. Schatzker classification of tibial plateau fractures: use of CT and MR imaging improves assessment. Radiographics 2009; 29(2): 585-97.
        [http://dx.doi.org/10.1148/rg.292085078] [PMID: 19325067]

[17]   Chen XZ, Liu CG, Chen Y, Wang LQ, Zhu QZ, Lin P. Arthroscopy-assisted surgery for tibial plateau fractures. Arthroscopy 2014.
        [PMID: 25125382]

[18]   Park S, Ahn J, Gee AO, Kuntz AF, Esterhai JL. Compartment syndrome in tibial fractures. J Orthop

Trauma 2009; 23(7): 514-8.
[http://dx.doi.org/10.1097/BOT.0b013e3181a2815a] [PMID: 19633461]

[19]   Chang YH, Tu YK, Yeh WL, Hsu RW. Tibial plateau fracture with compartment syndrome: a complication of higher incidence in Taiwan. Chang Gung Med J 2000; 23(3): 149-55.
[PMID: 15641218]

[20]   Stark E, Stucken C, Trainer G, Tornetta P III. Compartment syndrome in Schatzker type VI plateau fractures and medial condylar fracture-dislocations treated with temporary external fixation. J Orthop Trauma 2009; 23(7): 502-6.
[http://dx.doi.org/10.1097/BOT.0b013e3181a18235] [PMID: 19633459]

[21]   Adamson GJ, Wiss DA, Lowery GL, Peters CL. Type II floating knee: ipsilateral femoral and tibial fractures with intraarticular extension into the knee joint. J Orthop Trauma 1992; 6(3): 333-9.
[http://dx.doi.org/10.1097/00005131-199209000-00011] [PMID: 1403253]

[22]   Fraser RD, Hunter GA, Waddell JP. Ipsilateral fracture of the femur and tibia. J Bone Joint Surg Br 1978; 60-B(4): 510-5.
[PMID: 711798]

[23]   Milgrom C, Giladi M, Simkin A, *et al.* An analysis of the biomechanical mechanism of tibial stress fractures among Israeli infantry recruits. A prospective study. Clin Orthop Relat Res 1988; (231): 216-21.
[PMID: 3370876]

[24]   Maslov AV, Shcherbin LA, Mogutov SV, Shigeev VV. [Determination of the mechanical strength of the human crus to transverse directed impacts (bumper injuries)]. Sud Med Ekspert 1980; 23(1): 24-7. [Determination of the mechanical strength of the human crus to transverse directed impacts (bumper injuries)].
[PMID: 7355445]

[25]   Porter BB. Crush fractures of the lateral tibial table. Factors influencing the prognosis. J Bone Joint Surg Br 1970; 52(4): 676-87.
[PMID: 5487567]

[26]   Roberts JM. Fractures of the condyles of the tibia. An anatomical and clinical end-result study of one hundred cases. J Bone Joint Surg Am 1968; 50(8): 1505-21.
[PMID: 5722847]

[27]   Lansinger O, Bergman B, Körner L, Andersson GB. Tibial condylar fractures. A twenty-year follow-up. J Bone Joint Surg Am 1986; 68(1): 13-9.
[PMID: 3941115]

[28]   Ringus VM, Lemley FR, Hubbard DF, Wearden S, Jones DL. Lateral tibial plateau fracture depression as a predictor of lateral meniscus pathology. Orthopedics 2010; 33(2): 80-4.
[http://dx.doi.org/10.3928/01477447-20100104-05] [PMID: 20192139]

[29]   Biyani A, Reddy NS, Chaudhury J, Simison AJ, Klenerman L. The results of surgical management of displaced tibial plateau fractures in the elderly. Injury 1995; 26(5): 291-7.
[http://dx.doi.org/10.1016/0020-1383(95)00027-7] [PMID: 7649642]

[30]   Levy O, Salai M, Ganel A, Mazor J, Oran A, Horoszowski H. The operative results of tibial plateau

fractures in older patients: a long-term follow-up and review. Bull Hosp Jt Dis 1993; 53(1): 15-6.
[PMID: 8374484]

[31]   Caspari RB, Hutton PM, Whipple TL, Meyers JF. The role of arthroscopy in the management of tibial plateau fractures. Arthroscopy 1985; 1(2): 76-82.
[http://dx.doi.org/10.1016/S0749-8063(85)80035-9] [PMID: 4091921]

[32]   Gausewitz S, Hohl M. The significance of early motion in the treatment of tibial plateau fractures. Clin Orthop Relat Res 1986; (202): 135-8.
[PMID: 3955941]

[33]   Kennedy JC, Bailey WH. Experimental tibial-plateau fractures. Studies of the mechanism and a classification. J Bone Joint Surg Am 1968; 50(8): 1522-34.
[PMID: 5722848]

[34]   Delamarter RB, Hohl M, Hopp E Jr. Ligament injuries associated with tibial plateau fractures. Clin Orthop Relat Res 1990; (250): 226-33.
[PMID: 2293934]

[35]   El-Shazly M, Saleh M. Displacement of the common peroneal nerve associated with upper tibial fracture: implications for fine wire fixation. J Orthop Trauma 2002; 16(3): 204-7.
[http://dx.doi.org/10.1097/00005131-200203000-00012] [PMID: 11880786]

[36]   Wilppula E, Bakalim G. Ligamentous tear concomitant with tibial condylar fracture. Acta Orthop Scand 1972; 43(4): 292-300.
[http://dx.doi.org/10.3109/17453677208991267] [PMID: 4651050]

[37]   Colletti P, Greenberg H, Terk MR. MR findings in patients with acute tibial plateau fractures. Comput Med Imaging Graph 1996; 20(5): 389-94.
[http://dx.doi.org/10.1016/S0895-6111(96)00054-7] [PMID: 9007366]

[38]   Barrow BA, Fajman WA, Parker LM, Albert MJ, Drvaric DM, Hudson TM. Tibial plateau fractures: evaluation with MR imaging. Radiographics 1994; 14(3): 553-9.
[http://dx.doi.org/10.1148/radiographics.14.3.8066271] [PMID: 8066271]

CHAPTER 2

Tibial Plateau Fractures: Applied Anatomy and Classification

Luigi Sabatini[1,*] and **Wael Salama**[2]

[1] *University of Turin, Unit of Orthopaedics and Traumatology, Hospital San Luigi Gonzaga, Orbassano (Turin), Italy*

[2] *Orthopaedic Department, Sohag University Hospital (SUH), Sohag, Egypt*

Abstract: The tibial plateau fractures classification is very important for the clinical prognosis and to plan time and needs for surgery; however, the features of this type of lesion are various, and many classification systems were developed to describe variables that contribute to lesion pattern. It is also important the evaluation of soft tissues that are often involved (compartimental syndrome, exposition), associated knee injuries (meniscal or ligamentous), and general health condition in poly-traumatized patients. The AO/OTA fracture classification system is used by The Orthopaedic Trauma Association as for other fractures. Many surgeons prefer the classification described by Schatzker *et al.* because it is simpler and more familiar. Despite that there is limited inter and intraobserver reliability for Schatzker and AO classifications; future classification systems or revisions of the previous ones will have to consider axial imaging to describe in a better way the fracture patterns.

Keywords: AO classification, Schatzker classification, Tibial plateau fractures classification, Schatzker classification, Tibial plateau anatomy.

INTRODUCTION

As for all site fractures, when we manage tibial plateau injuries we have to evaluate the features of the fracture, associated lesions and possible complications. When we talk about intra articular fractures, the goals of treatment

---

* **Correspondence author Luigi Sabatini:** University of Turin, Hospital San Luigi Gonzaga, Regione Gonzole 10, 10043 - Orbassano (Turin), Italy; Tel: +39.011.9026619; E-mail: luigisabatini.ort@gmail.com

include achieving a stable fracture and an anatomic reduction of the joint surface, in order to preserve a functional ROM without need of immobilization after surgery. This result is important also for tibial plateau fractures; despite good anatomic reduction, we can see the development of a post-traumatic arthritis as well, due to the chondral surface injury.

An anatomic, stable reduction can avoid post-traumatic knee arthritis. Tibial plateau fractures may have different patterns, from undisplaced closed injuries treated with no weight bearing, to complex displaced fractures with diaphyseal extension and often soft tissue or neurovascular associated injuries that can affect the lower limb [1]. The fractures of the tibial plateau can involve the articular surface alone or, in more severe injuries, the metaphysis and diaphysis too. At the same time lesions of the tibial spines, tibial tuberosity, menisci and/or ligamentous structures can also be associated. The treatment of the fracture in these types of lesion should be more difficult. Classification systems can help surgeons to understand and treat these types of fractures in order to improve clinical outcomes. In addition, classifications are important for fracture prognosis and for communication between various surgeons when they compare and analyse these injuries.

APPLIED ANATOMY

An optimal knowledge of the site anatomy is important to understand better the fracture pattern and to plan the best treatment for the fracture itself and for the associated lesions. In the proximal tibia the intercondylar tibial eminences are between medial and lateral tibial plateaus. The medial plateau is the biggest one: it is concave in all spazial plane and has an articular cartilage surface thinner than the lateral plateau. This plateau, however, is convex in the sagittal plane and almost flat to slightly convex in the coronal plane. An angle of approximately 3 degrees of varus is formed by the tibial plateau with the long axis of the tibia, so the lateral plateau results slightly higher than the medial one. With a good knowledge of the tibial plateau anatomy, a wrong subcondral or intra-articular screws positioning can be avoided. The tibial spines are a non articular part of the tibial plateau and they are the insertion of anterior and posterior cruciate ligamentous. The footprint of the anterior cruciate ligament (ACL) is more lateral and anterior to the anterior tibial spine.

This area can be multi-fragmentated in high-energy injuries, and although this part is not articular it is important to restore the intercondylar eminence and the anatomy of the proximal epiphysis.

In the knee, the trabecular bone on the medial tibial condyle is stronger than the lateral one because load is predominat in this portion; for this reason a lower energy trauma is sufficient to cause fractures on the lateral side [2]. The intra-articular space between the femoral condyles and tibial plateaus is lied by menisci that are semilunar and triangular-shaped fibrocartilage. It is important to know their normal anatomy because they are often damaged or detached after trauma and we have to repair them during the treatment of tibial plateau fractures. The lateral meniscus is larger than the medial one and covers a larger rate of the lateral plateau. They protect the articular cartilage decreasing from up to 60% on the knee during weight bearing [3]. The anterior horns of these two structures are connected by the intermeniscal ligament and are attached peripherally by the coronary ligaments to the tibial plateaus. In addition, the anterior horn of the lateral meniscus is attached slightly posterior than the medial meniscus.

CLASSIFICATION

History

Palmer in 1951 [4], Hohl and Luck in 1956, and Hohl in 1967 [5] began to classify tibial plateau fractures; they already recognized the major patterns that are today the same for many classification systems for these fractures such as condylar split , subchondral depression, and comminuted bicondylar involvement. Schatzker *et al.* published their classification system in 1979, evaluating the AP radiographs of a series of 94 patients, most of them treated non operatively [6]. Schatzker classification divided tibial plateau fractures into six types: lateral tibial plateau split fracture (Type I), split depression of the lateral tibial plateau (Type II), central depression of the lateral plateau (Type III), split of the medial tibial plateau (Type IV), bicondylar tibial plateau fracture (Type V), and dissociation between the metaphysis and diaphysis (Type VI). The first three types involve only the lateral tibial plateau, Type III (depression) fractures are caused by low-energy trauma, often in osteopenic bone, the other types result from high-energy injuries [6]. Types IV to VI often result from road accident or falls from height [7].

The first four types are fractures involving one condyle while Types V and VI are bicondylar. Schatzker classification system was based on fracture pattern and each fracture feature is important to choose the appropriate surgical treatment, such as lag screws, buttress plates, one or even two plates as often is used for bicondylar fractures;

The classification underlines the importance of depression and the need of treatment to elevate the depressed joint surface; in many cases it is necessary to maintain reduction of depressed fragment with bone graft. Schatzker *et al.* noted in their series that fractures treated whit surgery had better results than those treated non operatively and that osteoporotic bone obtained worse results in both operative and nonoperative treatment [6]. Schatzker classification system was used in the past and it is used also today. In the following years other classifications tried to define these fractures in a more complete way.

Classification Systems

Nowadays there is no universally accepted method to categorize tibial plateau fractures; more than six classifications have been described in the past. Epidemiologists categorize these fractures in two lesion groups: higher energy injuries in younger people and lower-energy lesions in elderly patients due to osteopenia [8]. Two classifications are the most commonly used systems for describing such fractures, the Schatzker and AO/OTA.

Comprehensive anatomic classifications such as the AO classification or the Orthopaedic Trauma Association classification can be appropriate for research purposes (Fig. **1**) but they may be more difficult to use in sharing information between surgeons. Instead, the Schatzker classification is commonly used in the clinical practice. (Fig. **2**) [9]. Because of its simplicity if compared with comprehensive classifications.

In the Schatzker classification, a type I lesion is a "pure" split fracture of the lateral tibial plateau, without plateau depression. It is seen especially in young patients with strong cancellous bone and a peripheral tear of the lateral meniscus is usually associated in fracture with an important dislocation.

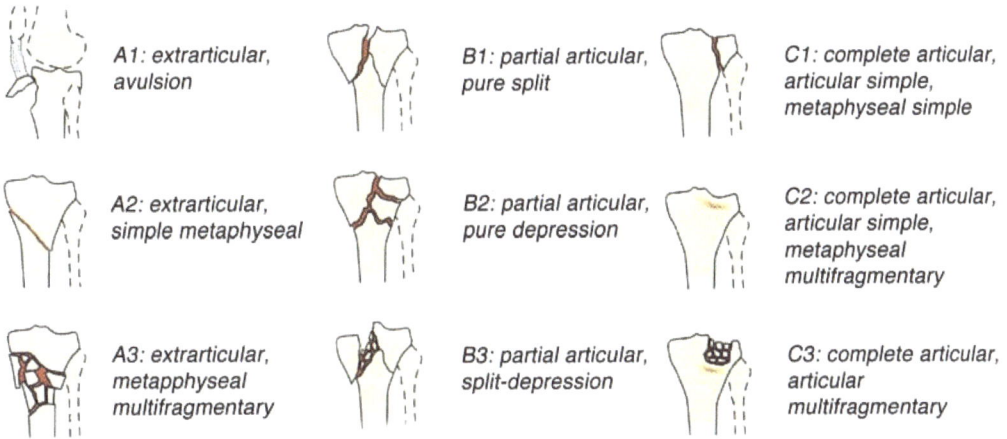

A1: extrarticular, avulsion

B1: partial articular, pure split

C1: complete articular, articular simple, metaphyseal simple

A2: extrarticular, simple metaphyseal

B2: partial articular, pure depression

C2: complete articular, articular simple, metaphyseal multifragmentary

A3: extrarticular, metapphyseal multifragmentary

B3: partial articular, split-depression

C3: complete articular, articular multifragmentary

Fig. (1). AO/OTA classification.

In Type II fractures there are split fractures of the lateral tibial plateau combined with depression. In the same way of type I injury, this type of lesion is often caused by a lateral bending force working in association with axial loading. Type III fractures are the most common fracture pattern in Schatzker's series (accounting for 36% of injuries): these are characterized by a pure depression of the lateral plateau, caused by low energy injuries, and for this reason more common in elderly patients with an osteoporotic bone; (Fig. **1** OTA/AO Classification) The type IV fractures involve the medial tibial plateau alone: because the medial plateau is stronger than the lateral one, they're due to high energy injuries and ligamentous/soft tissue injuries can be associated Type V injuries are bicondylar fractures involving both the medial and lateral plateaus, consequence of a pure axial load applied to a full extended knee, as it can happen to a driver involved in motor vehicle accident, who is pressing on the brake before the impact. Type VI injuries are the highest energy injuries and consists of fracture of the entire tibial plateau plus metaphyseal- diaphyseal dissociation. Using a classification system, orthopaedic surgeons can describe easily the grade of trauma energy (high *versus* low), the need for extensile or dual incisions in order to obtain a good reduction of the fractures involving both condyles or those with significant posterior damage, and the possibility of associated soft tissue injury. Split-depression fractures (Schatzker Types II and IV) present usually lateral meniscal and medial collateral ligament (MCL) lesions [10, 11]. (Fig.2 Schatzker Classification) Stark *et al.* distinguished in their series a compartment syndrome in eighteen per cent of patients with Type VI fractures [12].

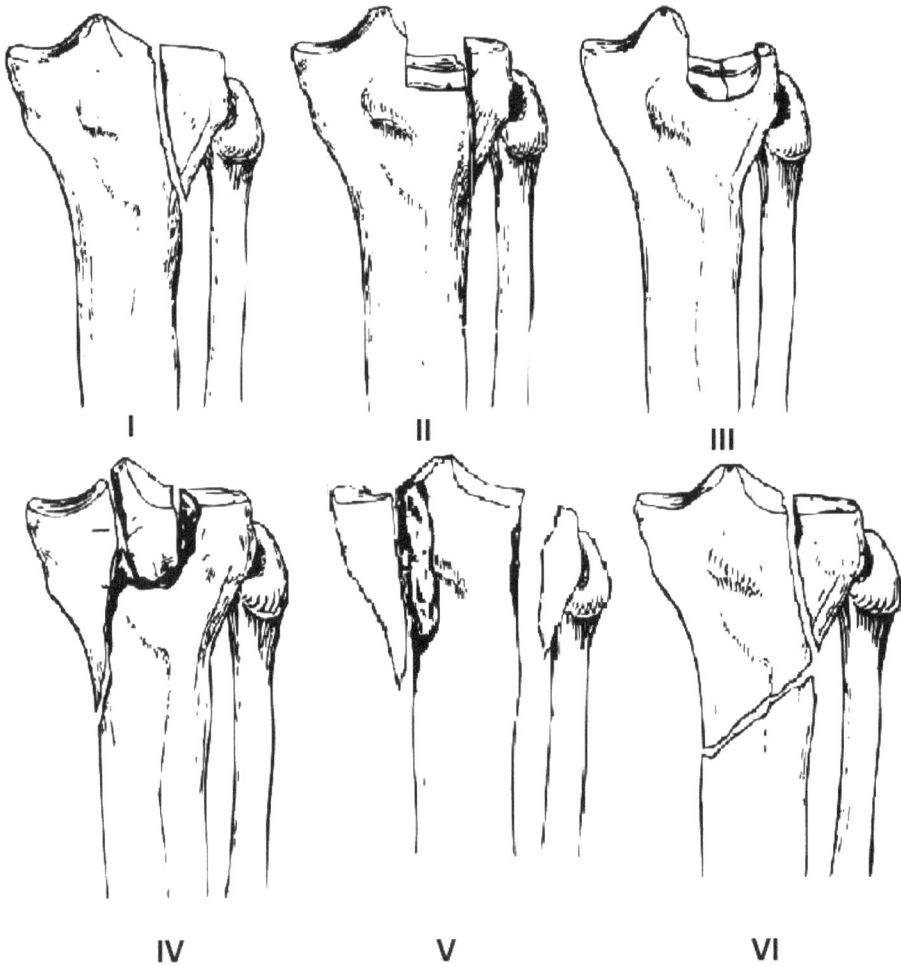

Fig. (2). Schatzker classification.

Type IV or medial plateau fractures are often thought as a consequence to transient knee dislocation events; for this reason these fractures require a careful neurovascular evaluation. The status of the soft tissues can be also evaluated with the Tscherne classification, an excellent system used by surgeons especially for closed fractures. Table **1** [13]. A grade 0 injury results from an indirect trauma and is associated with no soft tissue damages. A grade I injury usually results from low energy trauma and it is described by superficial abrasions or overlying contusions. In grade II injuries there are significant muscle contusion and possible deep contaminated abrasions: these can be the result of a bumper strike and are often associated with marked fracture comminution. The highest grade in the classification system is the third grade, associated with extensive crushing of soft tissues and subcutaneous degloving, with a possible concomitant arterial injury. In addition to the previous descriptions, patients who present incoming compartment syndrome automatically fall into the grade III category. Type of energy Type of lesions Grade I Low/moderate Abrasion, overlying contusions Grade II High Muscle contusion, deep contaminated abrasion Grade III High Extensive crushing, subcutaneous degloving, arterial injury. Compartment syndrome (Table **1** - Tscherne classification of soft tissue damage) Many Authors underline that there is an inter- and intra-observer difference when clinicians classify tibial plateau fractures using the Schatzker and AO/OTA classification systems. The Schatzker system was designed to classify fracture features with the use of radiographs alone, but when plain radiographs are used alone, studies demonstrate that intra and interobserver reliability is not so good [14]. Since CT has become very common for preoperative planning to analyse better the fracture features, several studies have evaluated its impact on interobserver and intraobserver reliability of the OTA/AO and the Schatzker classification. The results show that the addition of two dimensional (2-D) CT and three-dimensional (3-D) reconstructions of CT images raise the inter and intro-observer reproducibility to a satisfied level.

Table 1. Tscherne classification of soft tissue damage.

	Type of energy	Type of lesions
Grade I	Low/moderate	Abrasion, overlyng contusions
Grade II	High	Muscle contusion, deep contaminated abrasion
Grade III	High	Extensive crushing, subcutaneous degloving, arterial injury. Compartment syndrome

CONFLICT OF INTEREST

The author confirms that author has no conflict of interest to declare for this publication.

ACKNOWLEDGEMENTS

Declared none.

REFERENCES

[1]   Dirschl DR, Dawson PA. Injury severity assessment in tibial plateau fractures. Clin Orthop Relat Res 2004; (423): 85-92.
[http://dx.doi.org/10.1097/01.blo.0000132626.13539.4b] [PMID: 15232431]

[2]   Scott N. Insall & Scott Surgery of the knee. 2012.

[3]   Walker PS, Erkman MJ. The role of the menisci in force transmission across the knee. Clin Orthop Relat Res 1975; (109): 184-92.
[http://dx.doi.org/10.1097/00003086-197506000-00027] [PMID: 1173360]

[4]   Palmer I. Fractures of the upper end of the tibia. J Bone Joint Surg Br 1951; 33B(2): 160-6.
[PMID: 14832314]

[5]   Hohl M. Tibial condylar fractures. J Bone Joint Surg Am 1967; 49(7): 1455-67.
[PMID: 6053707]

[6]   Schatzker J, McBroom R, Bruce D. The tibial plateau fracture. The Toronto experience 1968--1975. Clin Orthop Relat Res 1979; (138): 94-104.
[PMID: 445923]

[7]   Barei DP, Nork SE, Mills WJ, Coles CP, Henley MB, Benirschke SK. Functional outcomes of severe bicondylar tibial plateau fractures treated with dual incisions and medial and lateral plates. J Bone Joint Surg Am 2006; 88(8): 1713-21.
[http://dx.doi.org/10.2106/JBJS.E.00907] [PMID: 16882892]

[8]   Zeltser DW, Leopold SS, Seth S, Leopold MD. Classifications in brief: Schatzker classification of tibial plateau fractures. Clin Orthop Relat Res 2013; 471(2): 371-4.
[http://dx.doi.org/10.1007/s11999-012-2451-z] [PMID: 22744206]

[9]   Schatzker J, McBroom R, Bruce D. The tibial plateau fracture. The Toronto experience 1968--1975. Clin Orthop Relat Res 1979; (138): 94-104.
[PMID: 445923]

[10]   Gardner MJ, Yacoubian S, Geller D, *et al.* Prediction of soft-tissue injuries in Schatzker II tibial plateau fractures based on measurements of plain radiographs. J Trauma 2006; 60(2): 319-23.
[http://dx.doi.org/10.1097/01.ta.0000203548.50829.92] [PMID: 16508489]

[11]   Bennett WF, Browner B. Tibial plateau fractures: a study of associated soft tissue injuries. J Orthop Trauma 1994; 8(3): 183-8.
[http://dx.doi.org/10.1097/00005131-199406000-00001] [PMID: 8027885]

[12]   Stark E, Stucken C, Trainer G, Tornetta P III. Compartment syndrome in Schatzker type VI plateau fractures and medial condylar fracture-dislocations treated with temporary external fixation. J Orthop Trauma 2009; 23(7): 502-6.
[http://dx.doi.org/10.1097/BOT.0b013e3181a18235] [PMID: 19633459]

[13]   Oesteren HJ, Tscherne H. Pathophysiology in classification of soft tissue injuries associated with fractures. In: Tscherne H, Gotzen L, Eds. Fractures with soft tissue injuries. New York: Springer-Verlag 1984; pp. 1-9.
[http://dx.doi.org/10.1007/978-3-642-69499-8_1]

[14]   Charalambous CP, Tryfonidis M, Alvi F, *et al.* Inter- and intra-observer variation of the Schatzker and AO/OTA classifications of tibial plateau fractures and a proposal of a new classification system. Ann R Coll Surg Engl 2007; 89(4): 400-4.
[http://dx.doi.org/10.1308/003588407X187667] [PMID: 17535620]

[15]   Brunner A, Horisberger M, Ulmar B, Hoffmann A, Babst R. Classification systems for tibial plateau fractures; does computed tomography scanning improve their reliability? Injury 2010; 41(2): 173-8.
[http://dx.doi.org/10.1016/j.injury.2009.08.016] [PMID: 19744652]

CHAPTER 3

Evaluation of Tibial Plateau Fractures: The Role of Imaging

Marco Busso*, Francesca Colonese, Federico Torre, Valeria Angelino and **Andrea Veltri**

University of Turin, Radiology Department, Hospital San Luigi Gonzaga, Orbassano (Turin), Italy

Abstract: Tibial plateau fractures are common injuries and the most difficult of the intra-articular fractures to manage. These fractures are usually related to high energy trauma or osteoporosis in older adults. The fractures normally occur in the 1% in older adults whereas in the elderly at 8%. In case of improper restoration of the plateau surface and the axis of the leg, these fractures could lead to development of premature osteoarthritis, injury in ligaments, as well lifelong pain and disability. The imaging is of paramount importance for assessment of the initial injury, planning management, prediction of prognosis and in the follow-up. Traditionally, the radiological examination was performed with x-rays. Presently, the computer tomography, affiliated with magnetic resonance imaging indicate more accurately the categories of fractures thus facilitating a better surgical plan.

Keywords: Computer tomography, Diagnosis, Imaging, Intra-articular fractures, Magnetic resonance imaging, Osteoporosis, Surgical, Tibial plateau fractures, Trauma, x-rays.

INTRODUCTION

Tibial plateau fractures are one of the commonest intra-articular fracturesresulting from indirect coronal or direct axial compressive forces. Use of technological progress in means of travel have resulted in a heightened number of accidents leading to incidents with complicated fractures.

* **Correspondence Author Marco Busso:** University of Turin, Radiology Department, Hospital San Luigi Gonzaga, Regione Gonzole 10, 10043, Orbassano (Turin), Italy; Tel: +39-011-9026401; E-mail: busso.marco@gmail.com

Those of tibial plateau are no exception. Being one of the major weight bearing joints of the body, fractures around it are of paramount importance. High energy trauma caused fractures are found in 1% of older adults and in the elderly at 8% rate [1, 2]. Tibial plateau fractures are often complex (estimates suggest that 30–35 % are bicondylar) and commonly occur with associated soft tissue injury [1, 2]. To date thediagnosis and management of complex tibial plateau fractures are acomplicated undertaking to resolve addressed in orthopedic trauma [2, 3]. As with any fracture, the aim of surgery is to restore the normal anatomy, repair soft tissue injuries, and facilitate the return to normal physiological functioning. In this context, the imaging has a central role for assessment of theprimary trauma, determining management and prediction of prognosis.

CLASSIFICATION

Fractures of the tibial plateau include a broad spectrum of fracture patterns. They encompass many and varied fracture configurations that involve the medial condyle (10-23%), lateral condyle (55-70%) or both (11-30%) with differing degrees of articular depression and displacement. A number of classification systems [4 - 10] have been designed to categorize and break down comprehension in clinical practice.

The OTA/AO system [8, 11], the Schatzker classification (Fig. **1**) [9] and the Hohl [5] classification are the systems mostly used in tibial plateau fracture assessment. Thus guidelines are issued for preoperative planning allowing for contrast and comparison in reported findings.

Actually, the fractures of the tibial plateau are typically characterized using the Schatzker system [9], in which fractures are classified as type I–VI. Each increasing numeric category specifies increased level of energy imparted to bone thereby increasing severity of fracture. First four are unicondylar and type V and VI are bicondylar.

In detail, type I is indicated by pure cleavage of the lateral plateau. Type I is found more so in 6% of all tibial plateau fractures in young subjects who have normal bone mineralization.

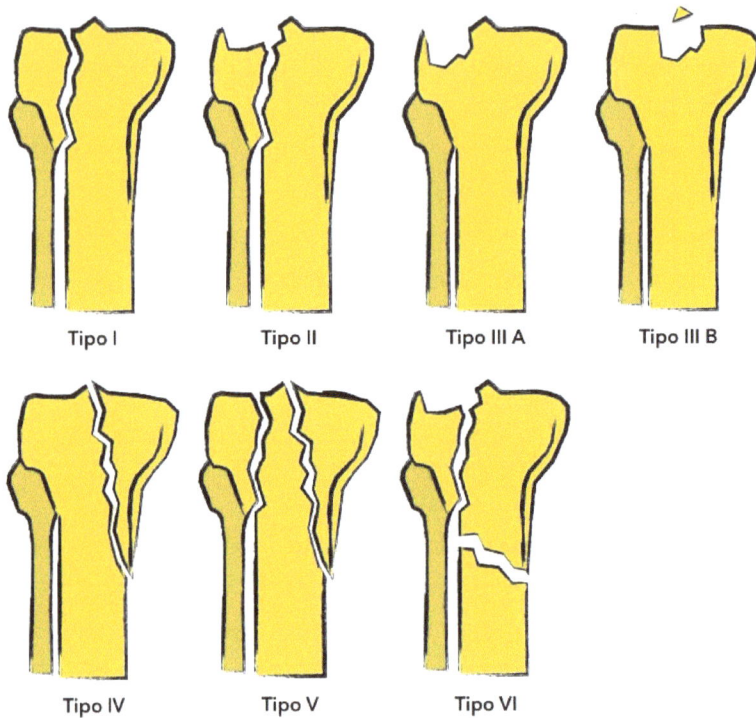

Fig. (1). The Schatzker classification.

Type II is characterized by a cleavage and compression fracture of the lateral tibial plateau, a type I fracture associated with a depressed component. They are found in 25% of all tibial plateau fractures and are notably common in patients in the 4th decade of life or older since a grade of osteopenia is necessary for depression to take place.

Type III is a compression fracture of the lateral tibial plateau in which the articular surface of the tibial plateau is depressed and driven into the lateral tibial metaphysis by axial forces. They are found in 36% of all tibial plateau fractures and typically in middle aged population (the 4th and 5th decades of life) with osteopenia.

Type IV is a medial tibial plateau fracture including a split or depressed part. About 10% of all tibial plateau fractures belongs to type IV category, and are effectively the most dire prognosis. These fractures are frequent in younger patients and related to high energy trauma. Type IV fractures from a low energy force can be sustained by older patients.

Type V is indicated by bicondylar fracture. They are normally linked to high energy mechanism injuries found for instance in automobile accidents and represent 3% of all tibial plateau fractures.

Type VI is indicated by unicondylar or bicondylar tibial plateau fracture with an extension separating the metaphysis and diaphysis. They stem from high energy knee injury representing 20% of all tibial plateau fractures. Each fracture's pattern in Schatzker classification helps to direct orthopedic surgeons to adopt appropriate treatment modality.

SURGERY

The treatment goal is to preserve normal knee function, so the orthopedic approach attempts to restore joint stability, alignment, and articular regularity to make certain a full range of motion. The approach of tibial plateau fractures can be non operative or operative. Non-operative method is a basic strategy that uses traction mobilization or functional cast bracing. However, the possible risk of complications related to prolonged traction or different types of immobilization should be taken into consideration, for instance decubitus ulcers, urinary tract infections, pneumonias, muscle atrophy, contractures, mental deterioration, leading to a prolonged hospital stay. The two major surgical techniques currently employed for tibial plateau fractures are open reduction and internal fixation (ORIF) and arthroscopic- assisted reduction and internal fixation (AARIF). Being less invasive, AARIF has a clear advantage over ORIF [12].

IMAGING DIAGNOSIS

Imaging is fundamental in order to diagnose precisely and then render appropriate surgical treatment for the patient.

X-Ray

Conventionally, tibial plateau fractures are classified using plain antero-posterior

(AP) and lateral plain radiographs [5, 9].

The standard views are the Anterior-Posterior (AP) and Lateral (Fig. **2**). In the context of trauma the lateral view is acquired with the patient lying supine and with a horizontal x-ray beam. In this way effusions can be visualised in the suprapatellar pouch.

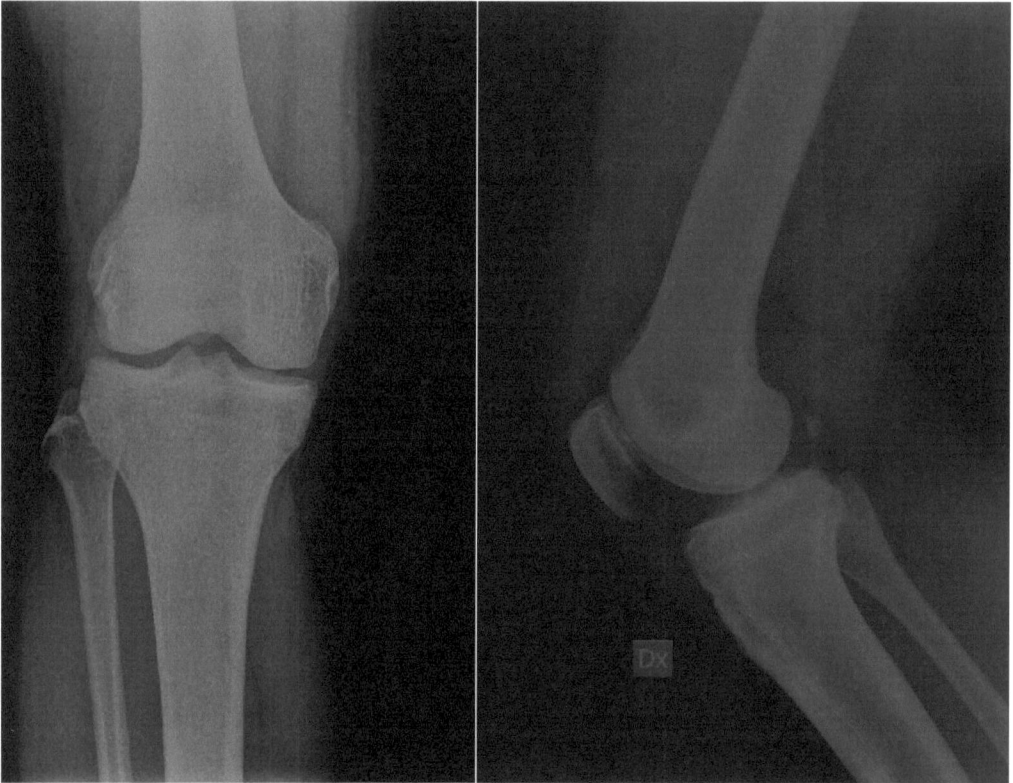

Fig. (2). The image shows anterior-posterior and lateral x-ray.

The Lateral view is feasible for evaluating soft tissues and bones. The quadriceps and patellar tendons are visible. The normal suprapatellar pouch between fat pads above the patella. Widening of these fat pads or augmented density in this area can indicate a knee joint effusion.

In the context of trauma, a 'Skyline' or 'Sunrise' view is rarely indicated. This view is only required in case of normal standard views associated with a suspect of a patellar fracture, or to assess patellar dislocation. Obviously, a skyline view can be acquired if the patient can tolerate knee flexion.

Some types of fractures can be detected exclusively by x-ray but there are many different pattern of fracture that are not represented in the traditional two-dimensional (2D) fracture classifications [13]. For instance, detection of a posteromedial fragment is relevant in preoperative assessment as it may necessitate an extra surgical procedure and/or extra fixation technique [14 - 17].

Moreover, posteromedial shear fractures, as well as fractures in the coronal plane, are frequently unseen on plain AP radiographs [16]. Even though there is a fast increase advancement in diagnostic imaging, the majority of studies evaluating reliability of characterization of tibial plateau fractures are set up on plain radiographs (Fig. **3**).

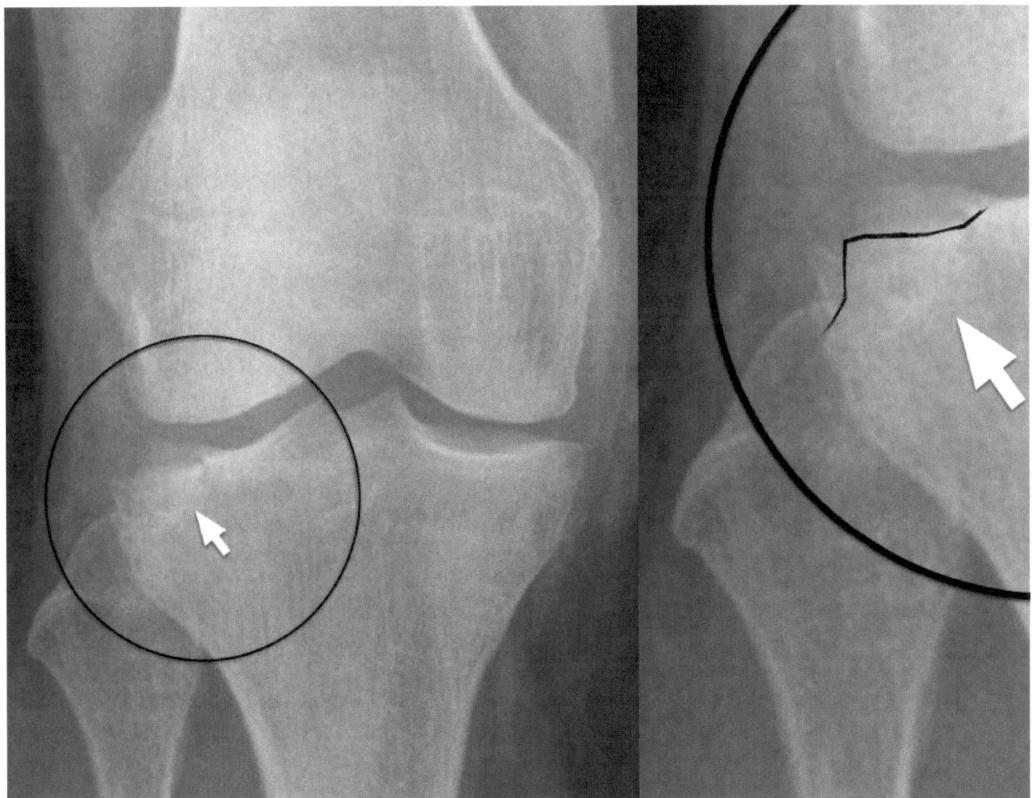

Fig. (3). Image shows depressed lateral plateau.

According to the intrinsic limits of the x-ray, the information given by the normal films is limited and does not completely support orthopedists in the diagnosis and treatment iter. Fractures of the tibial plateau, particularly complex fractures of the tibial plateau, need an additional assessment by computed tomography (CT) and magnetic resonance imaging (MRI). It has been indicated by various authors that baseline Schatzker rankings and surgical procedures based on plain radiographic images were changed after preoperative CT or MRI [18 - 20].

According to the Schatzker classification, we underline the difficulties in evaluating the fracture only with x-ray and as the MRI and CT imaging can improve the management of complex fractures [9, 21].

Type I fracture: as previously mentioned, it is characterized by a wedge-shaped pure cleavage fracture of the lateral tibial plateau, with less than 4 mm of depression or displacement. At plain radiography type I fractures could be slight. Depression could be not easy to evaluate on plain radiographs, and type I fractures can appear as type II fractures or *vice versa*. In addition, these fractures could be correlated with a distraction type trauma to the medial collateral ligament (MCL) or the anterior cruciate ligament (ACL).

Type II fracture: it is indicated by lateral splitting with depression. Depression cannot be well indicated on plain radiographs, and type II fractures can be similar to type I fractures. The measure of the depression is indicated by the vertical distance between the lowest point on the intact medial plateau and the lowest depressed lateral plateau fracture fragment, and originally it was defined exceeding 4 mm. The mechanism of trauma involves valgus force on the knee, distraction injuries to the MCL or medial meniscus and it is noted in 20% of the patients.

Type III fracture: it is indicated by pure depression of the lateral plateau. Depression may not be detected on plain radiographs. In addition, they are classified into 2 subtypes: type IIIA with lateral depression, and type IIIB with central depression. This subclassification is important since the surgical approach is different between the two groups.

Type IV fracture: is indicated by medial plateau fracture with or without an intercondylar fracture. They typically show a component of subluxation or dislocation, for this reason cross-sectional imaging can be more concise compared to standard radiography for evaluation of fracture extent. Furthermore, it is common a risk of compromisation of the popliteal artery and peroneal nerve. Finally, it is often linked to a distraction injury to the lateral compartment, leading to lateral collateral ligament (LCL) complex or posterolateral corner injury or in fracture or dislocation of the proximal fibula.

Type V fracture: fracture is composed of a wedge fracture of the medial and lateral tibial plateau, usually with an inverted "Y"aspect. Articular depression is generally appreciated in the lateral plateau, and there could be associated fracture of the intercondylar eminence. Type V fractures are dissimilar from type VI fracture patterns by the conservation of metaphyseal- diaphyseal integrity. Peripheral meniscal detachment are found in up to 50% of subjects with type V fractures. One-third present ACL avulsion injury. Condylar fractures cause instability by interrupting the support of the collateral ligaments. Further fracture of the intercondylar eminence is referred to as a four-part fracture and causes knee instability in consequence of loss of the cruciate ligament anchor. Cross-sectional imaging is generally used to rule out unstable four-part fractures.

Type VI fracture: the fracture is characterised by a transverse subcondylar fracture characterized by the separation of the metaphysis from the diaphysis. The fracture pattern of the condyles is various, and all types of fractures may take place. Soft-tissue injury are frequently associated.

Computed Tomography

A complete evaluation of tibial plateau fractures, must include a CT scan. Even though this is not mandatory for all tibial plateau fractures, it is fundamental in more complex fractures needing more precise information with respect to the detection and presence of split and depression areas or if the contralateral plateau has been injuried. CT, eventually associated to MRI, can be more concise in indicating the classification of fractures and bettering the surgical plan respect to x-rays [22].

It is extremely important to take into consideration the fracture depression and displacement since these factors may affect the surgical management. If untreated, depression leads to joint incongruity, valgus deformity, and instability. In case of displaced fractures, the meniscus could be torn and wedged into the fracture site, needing arthrotomy, disimpaction, and repair. These two factors are often mislead on plain radiographs, and cross-sectional imaging normally give more accurate details. For this reasons, in order to achieve an reliable estimation of fracture depression and displacement, CT is currently the conventional technique for preoperative assessment of bone damage. CT scanning is also recommended especially for comminuted cases [23].

Previous data have showed the reliability and reproducibility of different classifications under CT scanning and X- ray, and demonstrated the advantages of CT scanning [23, 24]. Data from previous studies have pointed out that surgical programs based on plain radiographic are revised in 6%–60% of cases after CT and 21% of cases after MRI [18 - 20].

The speed and availability of the TC render this technique valuable. Additionally, the majority of patients with extensive injuries inclusively go through CT of other portions of the body in the trauma setting. As a consequence, it has been estimated the efficacy of CT to detect soft-tissue damage. Gardner *et al.* [25] indicated that the dimension of depression and widening in type II fractures is predictive of soft-tissue damage. Depression superior to 6 mm or widening of superior to 5 mm augmented the likelihood of lateral meniscal injury (83% *vs* 50% in fractures with less displacement). Additionally, depression or widening of superior to 8 mm was correlated with an augmented prevalence of medial meniscal injury. According to these results, depression or displacement at plain radiography or CT may be predictive of soft-tissue injury.

Regarding the detection of ligamentous injuries at the CT scan, in the study of Mui *et al.* [26] CT and MRI were used to assess patients with tibial plateau fractures for detection of ligament tear and avulsions. Smooth visible ligament contours without obscuration by increased attenuation in adjacent soft tissues infer intact ligaments. CT showed torn ligaments with 80% sensitivity and 98% specificity. Exclusively 2% of ligaments believed uninjured at meticulous CT evaluation revealed partial or complete tears at MRI.

CT 3D

CT 3D reconstruction forms a perceptive image across the rotation and incision of the axis, that magnifies the identification of anatomical structures and pathological changes by showing several images from different spatial angles. This averts from the blind zone linked to vision limitations, hence bettering the diagnostic level and allowing for estimation of the degree of displacement of the fractures to be carried out in different planes.

It has been hypothesized an improvement in the intra– and inter- observer accuracy for the realization of tibial plateau fracture elements and classification through the inclusion of 3D reconstructions to 2D CT. Wicky *et al*. reported that by using Multi Planar Reconstructions (Fig. **4**) in tibial plateau management following 3D reconstruction, 59% of treatment plans were enhanced [18].

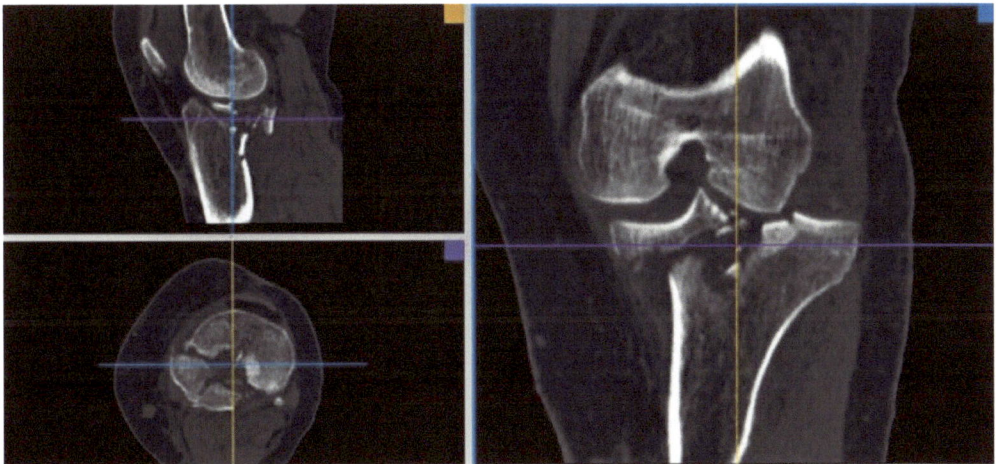

Fig. (4). The image shows Multi Planar Reconstruction CT (MPR) in complex tibial plateau fracture.

However, the reliability of its use was not investigated. Hu *et al*. [27] assessed the effect of 3D CT on the accuracy of classification systems for tibial plateau fractures. The results showed a better reliability with 3D CT in comparison with 2D CT in the assessment of tibial plateau fractures, but it was not reported if this was statistically significant. However, in the recent Doornberg study data [28], it can be seen that there is limited and non significant improvement in classification and characterization of tibial plateau fractures with the added use of 3D CT after

2D CT (Fig. **5**).

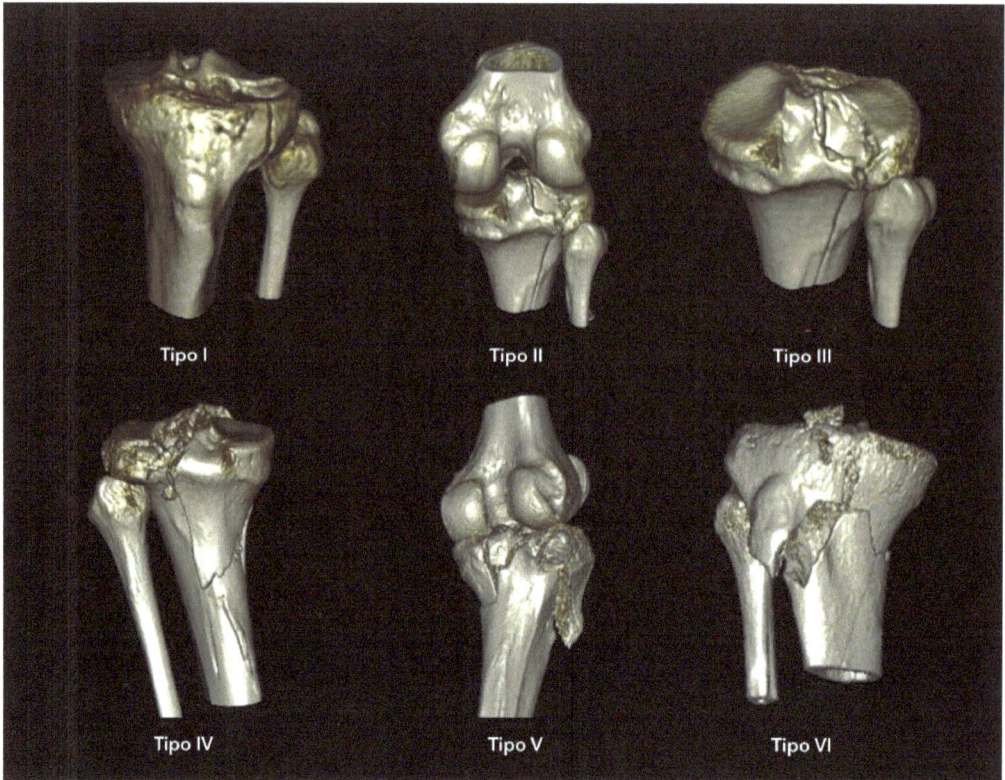

Fig. (5). The image shows Volume Rendering CT in Schatzker classification.

CT Angiography

Conventional angiography is being replaced by CT angiography for evaluation of peripheral vessels, also combined with CT for fracture assessment. In the event of any change in distal pulses or concerns about arterial injury, arteriography ought to be considered [29]. This technique should be used in the evaluation of high-energy trauma or for compartment associated syndrome.

Magnetic Resonance Imaging

Soft tissue management is a crucial problem in the treatment of high-energy tibia plateau fractures since soft tissues, particularly ACL, LCL, MCL and meniscus are often involved.

MRI is an additional study allowing a better detection of fractures and bone contusions around the knee joint and damage of the menisci and ligaments. Insidious fractures and bone contusions which cannot be diagnosed by the use of normal X ray films can be revealed with this method [30].

As well as for CT scan, surgical plans set up on plain radiographic images are changed in a relevant percentage of patients after MRI [18 - 20]. In the study of Yacoubian *et al.* [19], surgical findings in 54 cases indicated a 100% agreement with the MRI results of preoperative fracture assessment. In another previous study, MRI was found to be better or equivalent in determining degrees of fracture displacement when compared with CT assessment of tibial plateau fractures [31]. In order to understand if arthroscopy in diagnosis of cartilage injury could be substituted by MRI, Friemert *et al.* [32] evaluated 156 cartilage lesions arthroscopically detected with MRI findings. The end result that MRI is suitable for cartilage lesions exclusion is indicated by data reflecting an elevated specificity (97%–99%) and a negative predictive value (97%–98%) for cartilage damage. Regarding the soft tissue injuries, in the study of Gardner *et al.* [25] conducted in 103 subjects with all types of tibial plateau fractures, it was demonstrated an elevated percentage of disregarded injuries to soft tissues. No soft tissue injuries was seen in only 1% of the patients whereas total tear or avulsion of one or more cruciate or collateral ligaments was reflected in 77% and tears of one or more of the posterolateral corner structures of the knee appeared in 68%. MRI consent to rule out the majority of knee internal derangements effectively as established by the effective Crawford *et al.* systematic review [33] which focused on MRI arthroscopic and examination procedures.

Arthroscopy remains the most useful tool for managing menisco- ligamentous injuries even if it is an invasive procedure and may significantly increase surgical time. However, preoperative assessment with MRI could be valuable (Fig. **6**).

In the future, diagnostic image could be more useful in surgery, though the clinical significance of preoperative detection of meniscal and ligamentous damage currently remains unrevealed. Nowadays, orthopedists have acquired CT and MRI for preoperative evaluation of soft-tissue damage, particularly in case of a tibial plateau fracture.

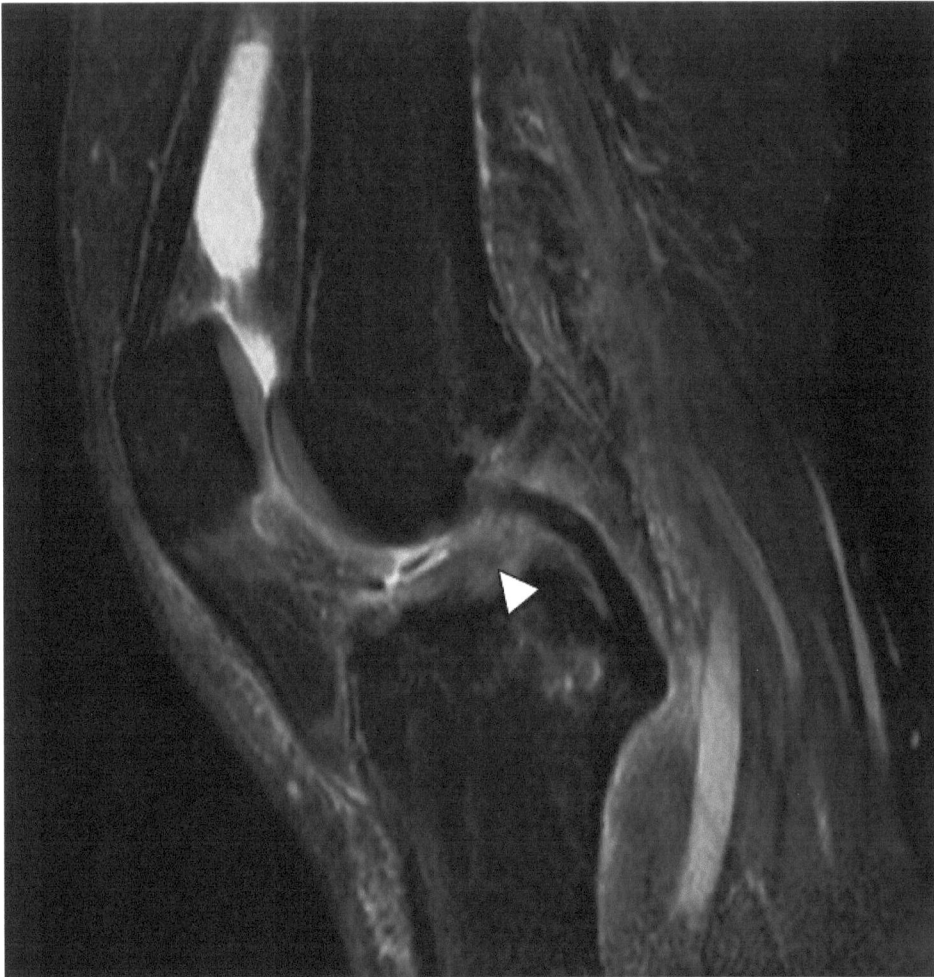

Fig. (6). Sagittal T2-weighted MR image shows an associated avulsion injury of the ACL [white arrow].

CONFLICT OF INTEREST

The author confirms that author has no conflict of interest to declare for this publication.

ACKNOWLEDGEMENTS

Declared none.

REFERENCES

[1] Thomas C, Athanasiov A, Wullschleger M, Schuetz M. Current concepts in tibial plateau fractures. Acta Chir Orthop Traumatol Cech 2009; 76(5): 363-73.
[PMID: 19912699]

[2] Burdin G. Arthroscopic management of tibial plateau fractures: surgical technique. Orthop Traumatol Surg Res 2013; 99(1) (Suppl.): S208-18.
[http://dx.doi.org/10.1016/j.otsr.2012.11.011] [PMID: 23347755]

[3] Asik M, Cetik O, Talu U, Sozen YV. Arthroscopy-assisted operative management of tibial plateau fractures. Knee Surg Sports Traumatol Arthrosc 2002; 10(6): 364-70.
[http://dx.doi.org/10.1007/s00167-002-0310-2] [PMID: 12444516]

[4] Charalambous CP, Tryfonidis M, Alvi F, *et al.* Inter- and intra-observer variation of the Schatzker and AO/OTA classifications of tibial plateau fractures and a proposal of a new classification system. Ann R Coll Surg Engl 2007; 89(4): 400-4.
[http://dx.doi.org/10.1308/003588407X187667] [PMID: 17535620]

[5] Hohl M. Tibial condylar fractures. J Bone Joint Surg Am 1967; 49(7): 1455-67.
[PMID: 6053707]

[6] Hohl M, Moore TM. Surgery of the musculoskeletal system. New York: Churchill Livingstone 1990.

[7] Moore TM. Fracture--dislocation of the knee. Clin Orthop Relat Res 1981; (156): 128-40.
[PMID: 7226641]

[8] Mu¨ller M, Nazarian S, Koch P, Schatzker J. The comprehensive classification of fractures of long bones. Berlin: Springer Verlag 1990; pp. 120-1.

[9] Schatzker J, McBroom R, Bruce D. The tibial plateau fracture. The Toronto experience 1968--1975. Clin Orthop Relat Res 1979; (138): 94-104.
[PMID: 445923]

[10] Wahlquist M, Iaguilli N, Ebraheim N, Levine J. Medial tibial plateau fractures: a new classification system. J Trauma 2007; 63(6): 1418-21.
[http://dx.doi.org/10.1097/TA.0b013e3181469df5] [PMID: 18212668]

[11] Marsh JL, Slongo TF, Agel J, *et al.* Fracture and dislocation classification compendium - 2007: Orthopaedic Trauma Association classification, database and outcomes committee. J Orthop Trauma 2007; 21(10) (Suppl.): S1-S133.
[http://dx.doi.org/10.1097/00005131-200711101-00001] [PMID: 18277234]

[12] Chen HW, Liu GD, Wu LJ. Clinical and radiological outcomes following arthroscopic-assisted management of tibial plateau fractures: a systematic review. Knee Surg Sports Traumatol Arthrosc 2015; 23(12): 3464-72.
[http://dx.doi.org/10.1007/s00167-014-3256-2] [PMID: 25246171]

[13] Eggli S, Hartel MJ, Kohl S, Haupt U, Exadaktylos AK, Roder C. Unstable bicondylar tibial plateau fractures: a clinical investigation. J Orthop Trauma 2008; 22(10): 673-9.
[http://dx.doi.org/10.1097/BOT.0b013e31818b1452] [PMID: 18978541]

[14] Bhattacharyya T, McCarty LP 3rd, Harris MB, *et al.* The posterior shearing tibial plateau fracture:

treatment and results *via* a posterior approach. J Orthop Trauma 2005; 19(5): 305-10.
[http://dx.doi.org/10.1097/BOT.0b013e31818b1452] [PMID: 15891538]

[15] Barei DP, O'Mara TJ, Taitsman LA, Dunbar RP, Nork SE. Frequency and fracture morphology of the posteromedial fragment in bicondylar tibial plateau fracture patterns. J Orthop Trauma 2008; 22(3): 176-82.
[http://dx.doi.org/10.1097/BOT.0b013e318169ef08] [PMID: 18317051]

[16] Weil YA, Gardner MJ, Boraiah S, Helfet DL, Lorich DG. Posteromedial supine approach for reduction and fixation of medial and bicondylar tibial plateau fractures. J Orthop Trauma 2008; 22(5): 357-62.
[http://dx.doi.org/10.1097/BOT.0b013e318168c72e] [PMID: 18448992]

[17] Galla M, Riemer C, Lobenhoffer P. Direct posterior approach for the treatment of posteromedial tibial head fractures. Oper Orthop Traumatol 2009; 21(1): 51-64.
[http://dx.doi.org/10.1007/s00064-009-1605-y] [PMID: 19326067]

[18] Wicky S, Blaser PF, Blanc CH, Leyvraz PF, Schnyder P, Meuli RA. Comparison between standard radiography and spiral CT with 3D reconstruction in the evaluation, classification and management of tibial plateau fractures. Eur Radiol 2000; 10(8): 1227-32.
[http://dx.doi.org/10.1007/s003300000326] [PMID: 10939479]

[19] Yacoubian SV, Nevins RT, Sallis JG, Potter HG, Lorich DG. Impact of MRI on treatment plan and fracture classification of tibial plateau fractures. J Orthop Trauma 2002; 16(9): 632-7.
[http://dx.doi.org/10.1097/00005131-200210000-00004] [PMID: 12368643]

[20] Macarini L, Murrone M, Marini S, Calbi R, Solarino M, Moretti B. Tibial plateau fractures: evaluation with multidetector-CT. Radiol Med (Torino) 2004; 108(5-6): 503-14.
[PMID: 15722996]

[21] Schatzker J. Compression in the surgical treatment of fractures of the tibia. Clin Orthop Relat Res 1974; (105): 220-39.
[PMID: 4609653]

[22] Markhardt BK, Gross JM, Monu JU. Schatzker classification of tibial plateau fractures: use of CT and MR imaging improves assessment. Radiographics 2009; 29(2): 585-97.
[http://dx.doi.org/10.1148/rg.292085078] [PMID: 19325067]

[23] Chan PS, Klimkiewicz JJ, Luchetti WT, *et al.* Impact of CT scan on treatment plan and fracture classification of tibial plateau fractures. J Orthop Trauma 1997; 11(7): 484-9.
[http://dx.doi.org/10.1097/00005131-199710000-00005] [PMID: 9334949]

[24] Brunner A, Horisberger M, Ulmar B, Hoffmann A, Babst R. Classification systems for tibial plateau fractures; does computed tomography scanning improve their reliability? Injury 2010; 41(2): 173-8.
[http://dx.doi.org/10.1016/j.injury.2009.08.016] [PMID: 19744652]

[25] Gardner MJ, Yacoubian S, Geller D, *et al.* Prediction of soft-tissue injuries in Schatzker II tibial plateau fractures based on measurements of plain radiographs. J Trauma 2006; 60(2): 319-23.
[http://dx.doi.org/10.1097/01.ta.0000203548.50829.92] [PMID: 16508489]

[26] Mui LW, Engelsohn E, Umans H. Comparison of CT and MRI in patients with tibial plateau fracture: can CT findings predict ligament tear or meniscal injury? Skeletal Radiol 2007; 36(2): 145-51.
[http://dx.doi.org/10.1007/s00256-006-0216-z] [PMID: 17136560]

[27]   Hu YL, Ye FG, Ji AY, Qiao GX, Liu HF. Three-dimensional computed tomography imaging increases the reliability of classification systems for tibial plateau fractures. Injury 2009; 40(12): 1282-5.
[http://dx.doi.org/10.1016/j.injury.2009.02.015] [PMID: 19535056]

[28]   Doornberg JN, Rademakers MV, van den Bekerom MP, *et al.* Two-dimensional and three-dimensional computed tomography for the classification and characterisation of tibial plateau fractures. Injury 2011; 42(12): 1416-25.
[http://dx.doi.org/10.1016/j.injury.2011.03.025] [PMID: 21570072]

[29]   Watson JT, Schatzker J. Tibial plateau fractures. In: Browner BD, Ed. Skeletal trauma: basic science, management, and reconstruction. 3rd ed. Philadelphia, Pa: Saunders 2003; pp. 2047-130.

[30]   Bencardino JT, Rosenberg ZS, Brown RR, Hassankhani A, Lustrin ES, Beltran J. Traumatic musculotendinous injuries of the knee: diagnosis with MR imaging. Radiographics 2000; 20(Spec No): S103-20.
[http://dx.doi.org/10.1148/radiographics.20.suppl_1.g00oc16s103] [PMID: 11046166]

[31]   Kode L, Lieberman JM, Motta AO, Wilber JH, Vasen A, Yagan R. Evaluation of tibial plateau fractures: efficacy of MR imaging compared with CT. AJR Am J Roentgenol 1994; 163(1): 141-7.
[http://dx.doi.org/10.2214/ajr.163.1.8010201] [PMID: 8010201]

[32]   Friemert B, Oberländer Y, Schwarz W, *et al.* Diagnosis of chondral lesions of the knee joint: can MRI replace arthroscopy? A prospective study. Knee Surg Sports Traumatol Arthrosc 2004; 12(1): 58-64.
[http://dx.doi.org/10.1007/s00167-003-0393-4] [PMID: 12904842]

[33]   Crawford R, Walley G, Bridgman S, Maffulli N. Magnetic resonance imaging *versus* arthroscopy in the diagnosis of knee pathology, concentrating on meniscal lesions and ACL tears: a systematic review. Br Med Bull 2007; 84: 5-23.
[http://dx.doi.org/10.1093/bmb/ldm022] [PMID: 17785279]

CHAPTER 4

Conservative Treatment of Tibial Plateau Fractures: Indications and Results

Jaswinder Singh[1,*] and Vivek Trikha[2]

[1] *Department of Orthopaedics, Indian Spinal Injuries Centre, Vasant Kunj, New Delhi 110070, India*

[2] *Department of Orthopaedics, JPN Apex Trauma Centre, All India Institute of Medical Sciences, New Delhi 110029, India*

Abstract: A force over tibial plateau with axial loading and valgus or varus vector can be responsible of tibial plateau fracture. The principles of management include joint congruity, joint stability, and axial alignment and the "personality" of the fracture. It is crucial to recognize, assess and monitor soft tissue swelling. In the present era, the indications for conservative management in form of traction or cast bracing are very few. Anatomical reduction is best achieved with operative modalities, either with closed or open techniques. However, non-operative modalities do hold their importance in certain situations like incomplete or undisplaced fractures, stable injuries, those with osteoporosis, and in patients who are not fit for surgery due to their medical comorbidities. Secondary articular cartilage injuries can be managed depending upon lesion size and activity demands, with simultaneous correction of malalignment and ligament instability wherever needed.

Keywords: Cartilage, Cast, Conservative, Injuries, Management, Nonoperative, Tibial plateau fractures.

INTRODUCTION

Bone fractures with articular involvement have been an important problem since past. Impairment was seen up to varying degrees. According to Charnley [1] in

* **Correspondence author Jaswinder Singh:** Department of Orthopaedics, Indian Spinal Injuries Centre, Vasant Kunj, New Delhi 110070, India; Tel: +917838128181; E-mail: hijaswinderin@yahoo.com

Francesco Atzori and Luigi Sabatini (Eds)

1961, anatomic reduction along with early mobilization were the preferred treatment for intra-articular fractures. These objectives were difficult to obtain because of the surgical and fixation techniques available in those times.

Pain, instability, malunion or nonunion were often result of surgery treatment. Greater stiffness was seen with surgery along with plaster immobilization, than plaster immobilization alone. Added surgical trauma and the periarticular location of the fixation device [2 - 4] was thought to be the cause of stiffness after surgery. Conservative treatment was so generally indicated for treatment of articular fractures and surgery was considered the last resort. Conservative treatment strategy included accurate evaluation, than fracture reduction and immobilization and finally rehabilitation. Joint stiffness was seen invariably during rehabilitation after fracture union. Apley encouraged early joint rehabilitation by "successful methods of traction to permit early motion of joints, while providing sufficient immobilization for the fracture union" [5, 6]. First results in tibial plateau fractures management with this technique were satisfactory, but not reproducible because tibial plateau fractures were not classified [6]. The new concepts by the AO group of atraumatic techniques of open reduction and internal fixation (ORIF) brought about a revolution in fracture surgery [4, 7 - 9]. However, with the increase in trauma energy (car accident, sport trauma), soft tissue injuries also increases. High-energy fracture types (Schatzker IV, V, and VI) were often treated with large surgical approaches and internal osteosynthesis through a tenuous soft tissue envelope. This led to high complication rates, with reported 50 percent in some studies [4, 10 - 15]. The time tested conservative treatment is now mainly indicated for stable and undisplaced tibial plateau fractures, or with fractures with excessive comminution, or advanced osteoporosis. It might be also the only treatment option available for a patient who is medically unfit for surgery. When chosen, near anatomical articular congruity should be attained along with normal alignment and early mobilization, to prevent compartment overload and future osteoarthrosis [16 - 19]. The concept of staged fixation is now favourable. With significant soft tissues compromise, immediate open surgical treatment can be dangerous. An external fixator initially can span through the zone of injury and overall limb realignment and stabilization is achieved. When the soft tissues have recovered sufficiently, "delayed fixation can be accomplished through a safe operative corridor of healthy tissues" [6].

INDICATIONS FOR CONSERVATIVE TREATMENT

Prognosis of proximal plateau injuries depend upon: (1) depth cartilage depression, (2) fracture fragmentation (3) fracture comminution and dissociation [3, 10, 20 - 25], and (4) extent of the soft tissue damage [21, 26 - 28]. Conservative treatment is indicated for low-energy undisplaced tibial plateau fracture or for stable lateral plateau fractures, and for some osteoporotic patients. Severe comorbidity of the patient can be a good indication for conservative treatment [6].

Instead, some authors state that articular cartilage depression from 4 to 10 mm is tolerable; depression over 10 mm is cause of instability and early osteoarthritis [5, 10, 13, 17, 22, 23, 29 - 40, 42]. Closed reduction (manipulation and traction) is not able to correct impacted articular fragments. Pauwels [41] demonstrated that "an incongruence of less than 1.5 mm appears to result in no significant increase in contact pressures". However, weight bearing increases stress rise in case of axial malalignment [42]. Mitchell and Shepard [43] showed that "malreduction and instability result in rapid articular cartilage degeneration". A correct reduction without contact over-pressure between femoral condyles and tibial plateau is an important factor for long term prognosis [22, 36]. Rasmussen [4] showed a "high correlation between post-traumatic osteoarthrosis and residual condylar widening or discontinuity between the tibial plateau surfaces and the femoral condyles".

The radiographic aspect of osteoarthritis does not always correlate with the clinical state [17]; however, it's fundamental to achieve anatomical reduction and stability to prevent compartment overload by correcting any coexistent axial malalignment.

Kettlekamp and co-workers suggested that "a major factor in determining functional outcome is the maintenance of the correct mechanical axis at the knee. A decrease in joint surface area and a rise in stress resulting from the deformity and the increase in axial loading may lead to post-traumatic osteoarthrosis" [16, 18, 32]. Sometimes, in case of high energy fracture, anatomic joint reconstruction is impossible to achieve If the metaphyseal and diaphyseal components are maintained aligned to mechanical axis, a reasonable functional outcome could be expected [54].

Schatzker and McBroom's review [9] has underlined some principles of treatment. Conservative treatment in a plaster cast for 1 month or longer caused marked stiffness of the knee. Open reduction and internal surgical fixation, followed by postoperative plaster immobilization, produced much greater stiffness of the involved knee [44]. So, intra-articular fractures, regardless of treatment, must be mobilized as soon as possible. In case of conservative treatment, "the joint with an intra-articular fracture should be treated with skeletal traction and early motion to preserve mobility" [2, 45, 46]. In this way, secondary joint surgical procedures (total knee arthroplasty or corrective osteotomies or cartilage regeneration) are usually more successful in case of good articular range of motion [47 - 51].

Conservative management of tibial plateau fractures still does hold its importance as surgical treatment of do not always guarantee perfect results. In a study of return to career in alpine skiers after they sustained a tibial plateau fracture, a large percentage of skiers with surgically treated intra-articular tibial plateau fractures could not continue to participate in downhill skiing; however, the majority could resume an active lifestyle for several years after the trauma. Fracture type seems to be an important factor influencing physical activity and general functional outcome [52, 53]. A fracture is considered stable if varus-valgus stress is minor than 10°at any point from complete extension to 90° of flexion. In case of partial articular tibial plateau fracture with wedge fragment, varus-valgus stress can be negative; this fracture pattern needs however anatomical surgical reduction and internal osteoshyntesis for sagittal instability risk [22] (Fig. **1**).

The absolute contraindications for conservative treatment are: (1) open fracture, (2) associated lesions (acute compartment syndrome, acute arterial injury). Relative contraindication is displaced tibial plateau fracture in a multiply injured patient [55 - 59].

Associated ligament injuries need usually surgical reconstruction [16, 60 - 67], but this argument is discussed in another chapter of this book.

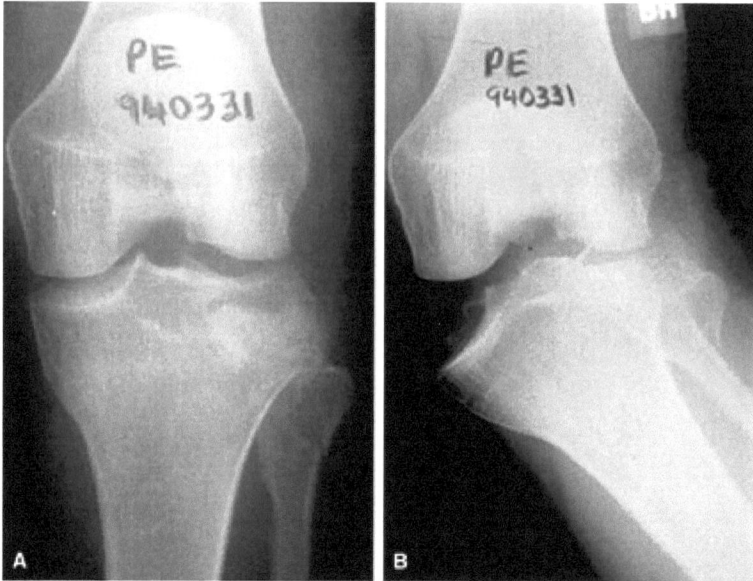

Fig. (1). Stress radiographs relevance. Valgus stress greater than 7-10 degree is indication for surgery. A, Lateral tibial plateau fracture in antero-posterior x-ray view. B, The same knee in stress x-ray.

CONSERVATIVE MANAGEMENT

Undisplaced and stable fractures are best treated non-operatively. Conservative treatment of these fractures needs early recovery of range of motion to prevent displacement [44, 57, 68]. Usually, hinged knee fracture brace is used to avoid secondary displacement and to permit motion [22, 44, 46, 65, 69 - 71] . In most instances weight-bearing is not allowed. Depending on fracture "personality", the knee is locked in full extension for 7-14 days. After 2 weeks, controlled passive range of motion will be increased, as though isometric quadriceps strength exercises.

The goal is to arrive at least 90° of knee flexion by 30 days after injury. Partial weight bearing is allowed with first radiographic appearance of consolidation. Weight bearing is progressed by 50% by 6 to 8 weeks and 100% by 12 weeks. If the radiological reduction is lost, operative treatment is considered.

A long leg cast can be considered for an unreliable patient who cannot be trusted to partial weight bear. The cast should be applied with the knee flexed to 45 degrees in this instance. Quadriceps atrophy and knee stiffness might the result with such a treatment due to prolonged immobilization [2, 72].

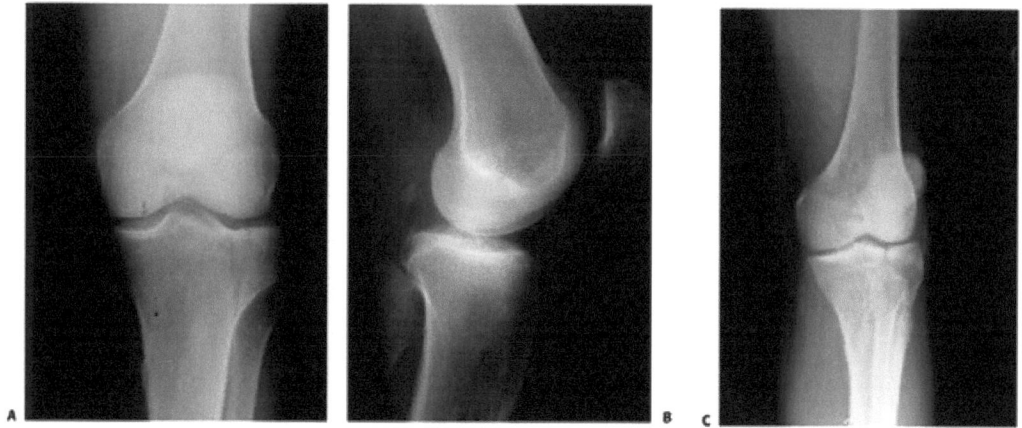

Fig. (2). A to C. Follow-up films of patient who returned to full activities, including marshal arts following a successful conservative treatment with protected weight bearing in a hinged brace.

In case of fracture comminution, important osteoporosis, or other patient-related factors, skeletal traction and early motion have to be evaluated. The historic management with only traction also still holds its importance; usually a distal supramalleolar tibial pin is used with 10 to 15 pounds of traction for indirect reduction by ligamentotaxis. Thomas splint and Pierson knee attachment can often be used to initiate early active knee flexion [2, 45, 46, 75] (Fig. **2**). X-ray control is obtained at 4 to 6 weeks after trauma: in case of initial consolidation and fracture reduction retention, the traction pin is removed and orthopedic brace is positioned.

Inadequate reduction of the articular surface as well as ineffective limb alignment control are the major limitations [73]. Furthermore, the extended period of hospitalization and recumbency should be avoided in today's health care environment. [22, 36, 61, 76]. Therefore, wherever needed, a staged treatment [73, 74] with early external fixation for soft tissue management, and followed by definitive fixation for high energy fractures is a standard protocol as per present literature.

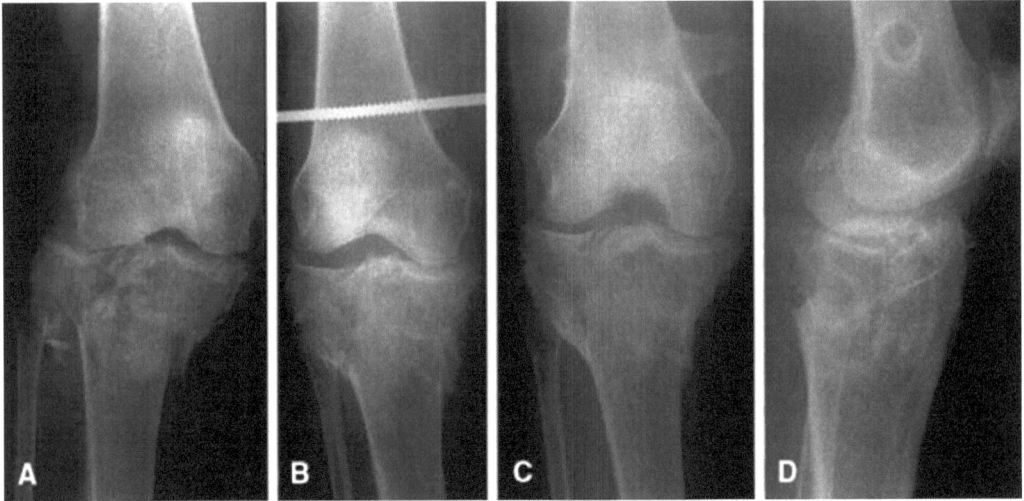

Fig. (3). A, Bicondylar fracture in an elderly patient with associated medical problems B, Conservative reduction. C, D, Control at 10 weeks.

Gausewitz and Hohl reviewed 112 tibial plateau fractures and found that "nondisplaced fractures or displaced fractures that were treated non-operatively regained preinjury knee motion even when immobilized for up to 6 weeks. However, fractures that were treated operatively developed significant stiffness with only 2 weeks of immobilization" [44]. Early mobilization is fundamental as it causes beneficial healing effects on the cartilage [77, 78].

Schatzker type II fracture (split-depression) is common in elderly population and this fracture is considered as stable fracture [10, 45, 46, 61, 76, 79, 80]. Opposite, Schatzker type IV and VI are unstable fractures and non-operative treatment in elderly population is usually adverse [61].

Luria and co-workers presented three cases of false negative x-rays in elderly patients with knee pain. The authors recommended "further diagnostic imaging with bone scan, MRI, or CT for patients that present with acute onset of knee pain and no trauma to rule out medial tibial plateau insufficiency fracture. The differential diagnosis includes osteoarthritis and spontaneous osteonecrosis". The three patients in their series were all successfully treated with conservative treatment as well as medical management for osteoporosis [81, 82, 94].

RESULTS

In 1990, Jensen and colleagues compared conservative with surgical treatment of tibial plateau fractures in more than 100 patients. Follow up was for 70 months in average. Meniscectomy was performed in more than half of the surgical patients. Though immobilization and duration of hospital stay were clearly shorter after surgery (P< 0.0001), the functional results were much the same. It was concluded that conservative treatment is a valid alternative to treatment to surgery, but should be reserved for cases where surgery was undesirable . The low frequency of osteoarthritis and of clinical instability and radiographic varus or valgus deformity indicate that fibrocartilage has good healing properties [24].

Sankhala and colleagues from India treated 75 tibial condylar fractures conservatively with traction and early mobilization. The period of follow up ranged from 6 months to 10 years; 89% (n=67) had satisfactory results. Stiffness, flexion deformity, osteoarthrithis and ligamentous instability were the major complications noted [97].

ARTICULAR CARTILAGE INJURIES AFTER TIBIAL PLATEAU FRACTURES

Articular cartilage healing is not possible even after minor trauma, though it can endure tremendous forces over many cycles. Hunter in his observation 250 years ago concluded that ulcerated cartilage once destroyed cannot be repaired. A viable articular cartilage is important for its health and function, otherwise arthritis develops: "in young athletic individuals usually traumatic articular cartilage changes are seen, whereas in older individuals, these changes are degenerative" [83].

Post-traumatic osteoarthritis incidence after tibial plateau fracture is different in literature and is due to articular incongruity and joint instability [17, 36, 84 - 86]. Decoster *et al*. reported radiological changes in 32% of patients at ten years follow-up [22]. In the follow-up of 106 cases, Jensen *et al*. reported 20% moderate to severe changes [24]. In his series of 260 fractures, Rasmussen reported 17% overall incidence of post- traumatic arthritis, with 42% in the bicondylar group [44]. Rademakers *et al*. showed 31% incidence of symptomatic osteoarthritis, which was more severe in cases with malalignment of more than 5 degrees [87]. Gaudinez *et al.* reported 83% of radiological changes in 1 year after comminuted tibial plateau fracture [55].

Symptomatically, articular cartilage injury patients present with pain, effusion, and mechanical symptoms. Usually pain is identified on medial or lateral knee compartment and worsen by weight-bearing and heavy activity; sometimes pain is accompanied by hemarthrosis and subchondral trabecular micro-fractures (bone bruises at magnetic resonance imaging (MRI)) [87 - 92]. Also for chondral lesion of the knee, traditional x-rays are needed: antero-posterior and latero-lateral weight bearing knee x-ray, Rosemberg view, patellar (Merchant or sunrise) view and bilateral standing hip-knee-ankle anteroposterior views. Then, it is fundamental to have a cartilage-sensitive MRI to classify cartilage injuries by lesion location, size, and grade (Table **1** and Table **2**). The lesion could further be well evaluated arthroscopically (Table **3**).

Table 1. Articular lesions classification by configuration (Bauer and Jackson).

Type	Configuration
I	Linear
II	Stellate
III	Flap
IV	Crater
V	Fibrillation
VI	Degrading

Table 2. Classification of articular cartilage lesions by severity.

Grade	Outerbridge	Modified Outerbridge	ICRS
0	Normal cartilage	Intact cartilage	Intact cartilage
I	Softening and swelling	Intact surface chondral softening or blistering	Superficial (soft indentation or superficial fissures and cracks)
II	Fragmentation and fissures in area less than 0.5 inch in diameter	Less than 50% of depth of cartilage with superficial ulceration, fibrillation, or fissuring	Lesion less than half the thickness of articular cartilage

(Table 2) contd.....

Grade	Outerbridge	Modified Outerbridge	ICRS
III	Fragmentation and fissures in area larger than 0.5 inch in diameter	More than 50%of cartilage with deep ulceration, fibrillation, fissuring, or chondral flap without exposed bone	Lesion more than half the thickness of articular cartilage
IV	Exposed subchondral bone	Full-thickness wear with exposed subchondral bone	Lesion extending to subchondral bone

Table 3. Articular lesions classification by configuration (Bauer and Jackson).

Fracture patterns		Bicondylar fractures	42%
		Medial plateau fractures	21%
		Lateral plateau fractures valgus	16%
			31%
Association with alignment after plateau fractures		Normal	13%

TREATMENT

Most of the studies done in the past for treating the articular injuries around the knee are based on age related cartilage lesions, rather than specifically for post-traumatic patients. Although epidemiology may differ, however, the treatment protocols for both the groups remain the same.

Treatment options for articular cartilage injuries and following arthritis can be non-operative or surgical options. Non-operative treatment includes decreasing the joint load, which include weight loss, activity alteration, and muscle strengthening across the joint. Other modalities include orthoses, braces and anti-inflammatory medications [93]. Surgical treatment is indicated for failure of non-operative strategy, to improve pain and mechanical symptoms. Different treatment options are described: debridement, marrow stimulation, transplantation to fill the defect, cell-based therapy, and the use of growth factors or pharmacological agents (Table **4**). The choice of procedure depends on "the size of the lesion" (Table **5**) and "the activity demands of the patient" [93].

Table 4. Treatment options for articular cartilage lesions.

Procedure	Indications	Outcome
Arthroscopic débridement and lavage	Minimal symptoms	Palliative

(Table 4) contd.....

Procedure	Indications	Outcome
Marrow stimulation	Smaller lesions, low-demand patient	Reparative
Osteochondral autograft	Smaller lesions, low- or high-demand patients	Restorative
Osteochondral allograft	Larger lesions with bone loss, low- or high-demand patients	Restorative
Autologous chondrocyte implantation	Small and large lesions with and without bone loss, high-demand patients	Restorative
Genetic engineering	Investigational	Restorative

Table 5. Operative reatment of articular cartilage lesions lesion.

Lesion Size	Operative Treatment
≤1 cm	Observation
	Abrasion chondroplasty
	Microfracture
	Osteochondral autograft transfer
1 cm-2 cm	Abrasion chondroplasty
	Microfracture
	Osteochondral autograft transfer
2 cm-3.5 cm	Fresh osteochondral allograft
	Autologous chondrocyte implantation
3.5 cm-10 cm	Autologous chondrocyte implantation
Multiple (2 or 3)	Autologous chondrocyte implantation

In small lesions (< 2 cm) and minimal symptoms in areas of limited weight bearing, arthroscopic debridement and joint lavage can provide short- term relief, reducing the inflammation and mechanical irritation. Debridement includes removing loose flaps, meniscal and osteophytes shaving and resection of inflamed synovium. Joint lavage reduces the synovitis and pain by removing fragments of cartilage and calcium phosphate crystals from the knee. These procedures provide "short-term temporary palliative effects, especially in older, low-demand patients" [94].

Abrasion chondroplasty or microfracture techniques (Fig. **4**) help in stimulating a reparative process for small lesions (<2 cm) in low-demand patients. They involve penetration of the avascular cartilage layer into the vascular subchondral bone to stimulate extrinsic repair. Symptomatic improvement has been reported in 60% to

70% of patients after abrasion or microfracture, but the result of fibrocartilaginous repair appears to deteriorate with time [95]. Gobbi *et al.* reported that despite initial improvement in approximately 70% of patients, at final average follow-up of 72 months, 80% reported a decline in sports activity level. In a study of 85 patients treated with microfractures [96], the technique showed simplicity of the low cost procedure and low risk of patient morbidity. Later patient may undergo other more complex procedures if needed.

Gill *et al.* [83] listed "various factors that affect the quality of the cartilaginous repair tissue after microfracture of a chondral defect: (1) during debridement, the abrasion of the subchondral bone must be avoided and only calcified cartilage layer must be removed, but; (2) a bridge of 1- to 2- mm of bone must be left between penetrations to allow connective tissue to fill the defect and adhere to the base of the defect; (3) Early use of continuous passive motion for joint function must be maintained after surgery; (4) depending on the location of the lesion, protected weight bearing must be strictly enforced; and (5) in conjunction with the microfracture procedure, any significant abnormality in the mechanical axis must be corrected" [83].

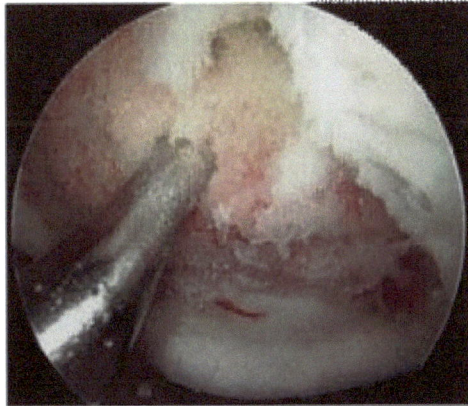

Fig. (4). Microfracture of articular cartilage lesion.

In high-demand patients with large or multiple lesions, restorative procedures such as osteochondral autograft transfer, osteochondral allografting, and autologous chondrocyte implantation usually are indicated.

Mosaicplasty includes transplantation of osteochondral autografts from portions of low weight bearing on the condyle as either a single large bone plug or multiple small plugs into damaged areas (up to 2 cm). Allografts can be obtained from a fresh osteoarticular size-matched hemicondyle for larger lesions (2 to 3.5 cm) [98 - 100].

Wilson and Jacobs [111] described an original surgical treatment for depressed comminuted fractures of the lateral condyle by removing the patella to replace the articular surface of the condyle. This kind of surgery is indicated only for fractures with extensive comminution. Jacobs reported his experience in 13 cases with satisfactory results with each knee being painless and stable, complete; though the flexion varied from 50 degrees to normal.

In another study of treatment of five severely comminuted bicondylar fractures of the tibia, Kumar *et al.* [112] described the use of a fibular head autograft. Excellent results were seen in three and good in one, without complications.

Autologous chondrocyte implantation can be an effective restorative procedure in lesions of 3.5 to 10 cm or for multiple lesions. This procedure involve two stages. In the first stage, autologous chondrocytes are grown from arthroscopically harvested articular cartilage or chondral bone. 3 to 6 weeks later a periosteal graft is sutured over the defect and chondrocytes are implanted into the chondral defect. Mechanical problems as malalignment, ligament instability, or meniscal lesions must be corrected before or at the time of autologous chondrocyte implantation. 80% to 89% patients have shown good and excellent results at 2 to 9 years after surgery [113 - 124].

87% success rate has been shown in 235 patients treated with autologous chondrocyte implantation by Minas and Chiu [123], and 91% good and excellent results has been reported in 112 patients by Gillogly *et al.* [118]. Arthrofibrosis (2%) and detachment (<1%) are the most common complications of this procedure.

In a study of 170 knees of which 97 required reoperation after autologous chondrocyte implantation, Henderson, Gui, and Lavigne, [121], found patch-related problems in 74% of those requiring reoperation earlier than 2 years, whereas cartilage- related problems 2 years after implantation.

Peterson [124] advocated an "autologous chondrocyte implantation sandwich technique" (Fig. **5**) to avoid multiple operative procedures. After filling the bone defect with cancellous bone graft, periosteum is sutured above the bone graft at the level of the subchondral bone. Chondrocytes are then injected between the membranes [125 - 127]. Bartlett *et al.* [113] described matrix-induced autologous chondrocyte implantation technique by utilizing porcine type I – type III membrane rather than periosteum [113, 114].

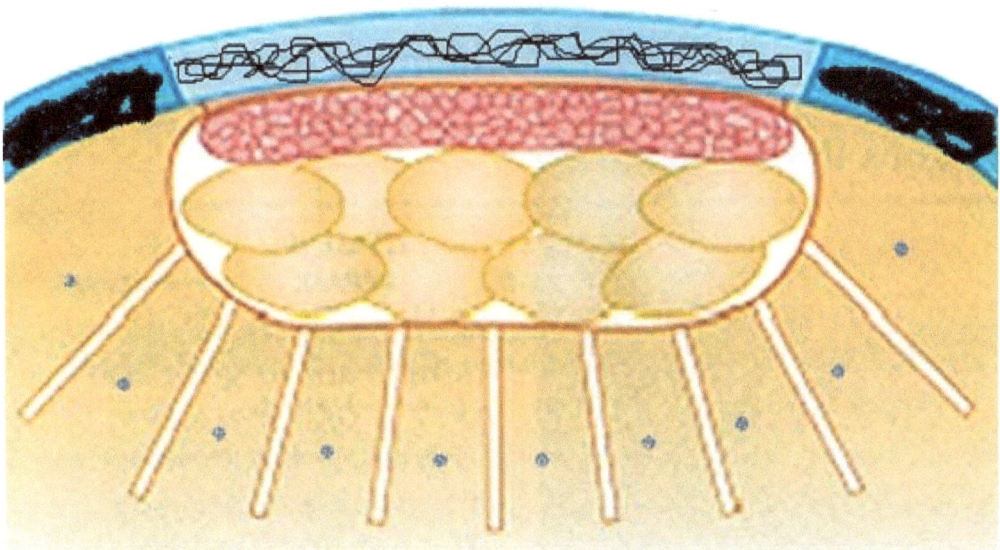

Fig. (5). "Sandwich" technique of autogenous chondrocyte implantation uses layers of transplanted bone, periosteal flap, chondrocytes, and periosteal flap.

Bioabsorbable collagen covers have been developed as an alternative, because of the frequency of periosteal hypertrophy and the difficulty of harvesting the periosteum and sewing it in place.

There is a concern about the uneven distribution of the chondrocytes in the defect and the possibility of cell leakage after the implantation of cultured chondrocytes in suspension. Biodegradable collagen-based [128] (Verigen, Leverkusen, Germany) or hyaluronan-based [129, 130] (Hyalograft C, Fidia Advanced Biopolymers, Abano Terme, Italy) scaffolds have been seeded directly with chondrocytes to avoid such problems.

Others scaffolds have been seeded with autologous chondrocytes inside a bioreactor for continuous hydrostatic pressure into the scaffold.

A constant disadvantage of autologous chondrocyte implantation is the long postoperative rehabilitation, with prolonged no-weight bearing and activity restrictions [127].

"Gene therapy" is a new method to carry genetic information to cells that contribute to the healing process. This strategy is being currently being developed to manipulate the repair process at the cellular and molecular levels. Ongoing research includes finding of an "efficient vector for delivering this genetic information and the candidate genes that are likely to improve cartilage repair and regeneration" [125 - 127].

CONFLICT OF INTEREST

The author confirms that author has no conflict of interest to declare for this publication.

ACKNOWLEDGEMENTS

Declared none.

REFERENCES

[1]   Charnley J. The Closed Treatment of Common Fractures. 3rd ed., Baltimore: Williams & Wilkins 1961.
        [http://dx.doi.org/10.1017/CBO9780511666520]

[2]   Hohl M, Luck JV. Fractures of the tibial condyle; a clinical and experimental study. J Bone Joint Surg Am 1956; 38-A(5): 1001-18.
        [PMID: 13367078]

[3]   Lachiewicz PF, Funcik T. Factors influencing the results of open reduction and internal fixation of tibial plateau fractures. Clin Orthop Relat Res 1990; (259): 210-5.
        [PMID: 2208858]

[4]   Waddell JP, Johnston DW, Neidre A. Fractures of the tibial plateau: a review of ninety-five patients and comparison of treatment methods. J Trauma 1981; 21(5): 376-81.
        [http://dx.doi.org/10.1097/00005373-198105000-00007] [PMID: 7230283]

[5]   Apley AG. Fractures of the tibial plateau. Orthop Clin North Am 1979; 10(1): 61-74.
        [PMID: 450404]

[6]   Bruce D, Alan M, Peter G, Christian Krettek. Skeletal trauma: basic science, management, and reconstruction. 4th ed., Elsevier: W. B Saunders 2009.

[7]   Barrett MO, Kazmier P, Anglen JO. Repair or reattachment of the meniscus after fixation of a tibial plateau fracture. J Orthop Trauma 2005; 19(3): 198-200.
[http://dx.doi.org/10.1097/00005131-200503000-00008] [PMID: 15758674]

[8]   Clancey GJ, Hansen ST Jr. Open fractures of the tibia: a review of one hundred and two cases. J Bone Joint Surg Am 1978; 60(1): 118-22.
[PMID: 624749]

[9]   Schatzker J, McBroom R, Bruce D. The tibial plateau fracture. The Toronto experience 1968--1975. Clin Orthop Relat Res 1979; (138): 94-104.
[PMID: 445923]

[10]   Moore TM, Patzakis MJ, Harvey JP. Tibial plateau fractures: definition, demographics, treatment rationale, and long-term results of closed traction management or operative reduction. J Orthop Trauma 1987; 1(2): 97-119.
[http://dx.doi.org/10.1097/00005131-198702010-00001] [PMID: 3333518]

[11]   Perry CR, Evans LG, Rice S, Fogarty J, Burdge RE. A new surgical approach to fractures of the lateral tibial plateau. J Bone Joint Surg Am 1984; 66(8): 1236-40.
[PMID: 6548477]

[12]   Savoie FH, Vander Griend RA, Ward EF, Hughes JL. Tibial plateau fractures. A review of operative treatment using AO technique. Orthopedics 1987; 10(5): 745-50.
[PMID: 3588420]

[13]   Schatzker J. Fractures of the tibial plateau. In: Schatzker J, Tile M, Eds. Rationale of Operative Fracture Care. Berlin: Springer-Verlag 1988; p. 279.

[14]   Stokel EA, Sadasivan KK. Tibial plateau fractures: standardized evaluation of operative results. Orthopedics 1991; 14(3): 263-70.
[PMID: 2020625]

[15]   Young MJ, Barrack RL. Complications of internal fixation of tibial plateau fractures. Orthop Rev 1994; 23(2): 149-54.
[PMID: 8196973]

[16]   Delamarter RB, Hohl M, Hopp E Jr. Ligament injuries associated with tibial plateau fractures. Clin Orthop Relat Res 1990; (250): 226-33.
[PMID: 2293934]

[17]   Honkonen SE. Degenerative arthritis after tibial plateau fractures. J Orthop Trauma 1995; 9(4): 273-7.
[http://dx.doi.org/10.1097/00005131-199509040-00001] [PMID: 7562147]

[18]   Houben PF, van der Linden ES, van den Wildenberg FA, Stapert JW. Functional and radiological outcome after intra-articular tibial plateau fractures. Injury 1997; 28(7): 459-62.
[http://dx.doi.org/10.1016/S0020-1383(97)00064-8] [PMID: 9509087]

[19]   Kettelkamp DB, Hillberry BM, Murrish DE, Heck DA. Degenerative arthritis of the knee secondary to fracture malunion. Clin Orthop Relat Res 1988; (234): 159-69.
[PMID: 3409571]

[20] Buchko GM, Johnson DH. Arthroscopy assisted operative management of tibial plateau fractures. Clin Orthop Relat Res 1996; (332): 29-36.
[http://dx.doi.org/10.1097/00003086-199611000-00006] [PMID: 8913143]

[21] Burri C, Bartzke G, Coldewey J, Muggler E. Fractures of the tibial plateau. Clin Orthop Relat Res 1979; (138): 84-93.
[PMID: 445922]

[22] DeCoster TA, Nepola JV, el-Khoury GY. Cast brace treatment of proximal tibia fractures. A ten-year follow-up study. Clin Orthop Relat Res 1988; (231): 196-204.
[PMID: 3370874]

[23] Honkonen SE, JAärvinen MJ. Classification of fractures of the tibial condyles. J Bone Joint Surg Br 1992; 74(6): 840-7.
[PMID: 1447244]

[24] Jensen DB, Rude C, Duus B, Bjerg-Nielsen A. Tibial plateau fractures. A comparison of conservative and surgical treatment. J Bone Joint Surg Br 1990; 72(1): 49-52.
[PMID: 2298794]

[25] Mallik AR, Covall DJ, Whitelaw GP. Internal *versus* external fixation of bicondylar tibial plateau fractures. Orthop Rev 1992; 21(12): 1433-6.
[PMID: 1465305]

[26] Fernandez DL. Anterior approach to the knee with osteotomy of the tibial tubercle for bicondylar tibial fractures. J Bone Joint Surg Am 1988; 70(2): 208-19.
[PMID: 3343265]

[27] Tscherne H, Gotzen L. Fractures With Soft Tissue Injuries. Berlin: Springer-Verlag 1984; pp. 1-166.
[http://dx.doi.org/10.1007/978-3-642-69499-8]

[28] Tscherne H, Lobenhoffer P. Tibial plateau fractures. Management and expected results. Clin Orthop Relat Res 1993; (292): 87-100.
[PMID: 8519141]

[29] Chan PS, Klimkiewicz JJ, Luchetti WT, *et al.* Impact of CT scan on treatment plan and fracture classification of tibial plateau fractures. J Orthop Trauma 1997; 11(7): 484-9.
[http://dx.doi.org/10.1097/00005131-199710000-00005] [PMID: 9334949]

[30] Hohl M. Tibial condylar fractures. J Bone Joint Surg Am 1967; 49(7): 1455-67.
[PMID: 6053707]

[31] Honkonen SE. Indications for surgical treatment of tibial condyle fractures. Clin Orthop Relat Res 1994; (302): 199-205.
[PMID: 8168301]

[32] Moore TM, Meyers MH, Harvey JP Jr. Collateral ligament laxity of the knee. Long-term comparison between plateau fractures and normal. J Bone Joint Surg Am 1976; 58(5): 594-8.
[PMID: 932058]

[33] Rangitsch MR, Duwelius PJ, Colville MR. Limited internal fixation of tibial plateau fractures. J Orthop Trauma 1993; 7: 168-9.
[http://dx.doi.org/10.1097/00005131-199304000-00045]

[34]   Segal D, Franchi AV, Campanile J. Iliac autograft for reconstruction of severely depressed fracture of a lateral tibial plateau. Brief note. J Bone Joint Surg Am 1985; 67(8): 1270-2.
[PMID: 3902847]

[35]   Reid JS, Van Slyke MA, Moulton MJ, Mann TA. Safe placement of proximal tibial transfixation wires with respect to intracapsular penetration. J Orthop Trauma 2001; 15(1): 10-7.
[http://dx.doi.org/10.1097/00005131-200101000-00003] [PMID: 11147682]

[36]   Lansinger O, Bergman B, KAärner L, Andersson GB. Tibial condylar fractures. A twenty-year follow-up. J Bone Joint Surg Am 1986; 68(1): 13-9.
[PMID: 3941115]

[37]   Rafii M, Lamont JG, Firooznia H. Tibial plateau fractures: CT evaluation and classification. Crit Rev Diagn Imaging 1987; 27(2): 91-112.
[PMID: 3608544]

[38]   Jennings JE. Arthroscopic management of tibial plateau fractures. Arthroscopy 1985; 1(3): 160-8.
[http://dx.doi.org/10.1016/S0749-8063(85)80003-7] [PMID: 4096767]

[39]   Kennedy JC, Bailey WH. Experimental tibial-plateau fractures. Studies of the mechanism and a classification. J Bone Joint Surg Am 1968; 50(8): 1522-34.
[PMID: 5722848]

[40]   Watson JT, Coufal C. Treatment of complex lateral plateau fractures using Ilizarov techniques. Clin Orthop Relat Res 1998; (353): 97-106.
[http://dx.doi.org/10.1097/00003086-199808000-00012] [PMID: 9728164]

[41]   Pauwels F. NeueRichtlinienfuer die operative Behandlung der Coxarthrose. VerhDtschOrthopGes 1932; 48: 332-6.

[42]   Brown TD, Anderson DD, Nepola JV, Singerman RJ, Pedersen DR, Brand RA. Contact stress aberrations following imprecise reduction of simple tibial plateau fractures. J Orthop Res 1988; 6(6): 851-62.
[http://dx.doi.org/10.1002/jor.1100060609] [PMID: 3171765]

[43]   Mitchell N, Shepard N. Healing of articular cartilage in intra-articular fractures in rabbits. J Bone Joint Surg Am 1980; 62(4): 628-34.
[PMID: 7380860]

[44]   Gausewitz S, Hohl M. The significance of early motion in the treatment of tibial plateau fractures. Clin Orthop Relat Res 1986; (202): 135-8.
[PMID: 3955941]

[45]   Rasmussen PS. Tibial condylar fractures. Impairment of knee joint stability as an indication for surgical treatment. J Bone Joint Surg Am 1973; 55(7): 1331-50.
[PMID: 4586086]

[46]   Marwah V, Gadegone WM, Magarkar DS. The treatment of fractures of the tibial plateau by skeletal traction and early mobilisation. Int Orthop 1985; 9(4): 217-21.
[http://dx.doi.org/10.1007/BF00266506] [PMID: 4093221]

[47]   Scotland T, Wardlaw D. The use of cast-bracing as treatment for fractures of the tibial plateau. J Bone Joint Surg Br 1981; 63B(4): 575-8.

[PMID: 7298688]

[48]   Prasad G, Zahn H. Medial tibial hemi-condylar elevation osteotomy as an operative technique to treat varus mal-united tibial plateau fracture. Musculoskelet Surg 2012; 96(1): 63-6.
[http://dx.doi.org/10.1007/s12306-011-0152-5] [PMID: 21773698]

[49]   Singh H, Singh VR, Yuvarajan P, Maini L, Gautam VK. Open wedge osteotomy of the proximal medial tibia for malunited tibial plateau fractures. J Orthop Surg (Hong Kong) 2011; 19(1): 57-9.
[PMID: 21519078]

[50]   Yu C, Yang M, Wang Z. [Reconstruction of malunited fracture of tibial plateau]. Zhongguo Xiu Fu Chong Jian Wai Ke Za Zhi 2007; 21(10): 1031-5.
[PMID: 17990763]

[51]   Saengnipanthkul S. Uni-condyle high tibial osteotomy for malunion of medial plateau fracture: surgical technique and case report. J Med Assoc Thai 2012; 95(12): 1619-24.
[PMID: 23390795]

[52]   Krettek C, Hawi N, Jagodzinski M. [Intracondylar segment osteotomy: correction of intra-articular malalignment after fracture of the tibial plateau]. Unfallchirurg 2013; 116(5): 413-26.
[http://dx.doi.org/10.1007/s00113-013-2377-2] [PMID: 23681487]

[53]   MA1/4ller D, Sandmann GH, MartetschlAã ger F, StAãckle U, Kraus TM. [Tibial plateau fractures in alpine skiing--return to the slopes or career end?]. Sportverletz Sportschaden 2014; 28(1): 24-30.
[PMID: 24665013]

[54]   Loibl M, BAãumlein M, Massen F, *et al.* Sports activity after surgical treatment of intra-articular tibial plateau fractures in skiers. Am J Sports Med 2013; 41(6): 1340-7.
[http://dx.doi.org/10.1177/0363546513489524] [PMID: 23733831]

[55]   Yong CK, Choon DS. Mid-term results of tibial plateau fractures. Med J Malaysia 2005; 60 (Suppl. C): 83-90.
[PMID: 16381290]

[56]   Gaudinez RF, Mallik AR, Szporn M. Hybrid external fixation of comminuted tibial plateau fractures. Clin Orthop Relat Res 1996; (328): 203-10.
[http://dx.doi.org/10.1097/00003086-199607000-00032] [PMID: 8653958]

[57]   Blaser PF, Wicky S, Husmann O, Meuli RA, Leyvraz PF. [Value of 3D CT in diagnosis and treatment of fractures of the tibial plateau]. Swiss Surg 1998; 4(4): 180-6.
[PMID: 9757807]

[58]   Chapman MW. The use of immediate internal fixation in open fractures. Orthop Clin North Am 1980; 11(3): 579-91.
[PMID: 6106173]

[59]   Edwards CC. Staged reconstruction of complex open tibial fractures using Hoffmann external fixation. Clinical decisions and dilemmas. Clin Orthop Relat Res 1983; (178): 130-61.
[PMID: 6349894]

[60]   Koval KJ, Helfet DL. Tibial plateau fractures: Evaluation and treatment. J Am Acad Orthop Surg 1995; 3(2): 86-94.
[PMID: 10790657]

[61] Mikulak SA, Gold SM, Zinar DM. Small wire external fixation of high energy tibial plateau fractures. Clin Orthop Relat Res 1998; (356): 230-8.
[http://dx.doi.org/10.1097/00003086-199811000-00031] [PMID: 9917689]

[62] Delamarter R, Hohl M. The cast brace and tibial plateau fractures. Clin Orthop Relat Res 1989; (242): 26-31.
[PMID: 2706855]

[63] Fowble CD, Zimmer JW, Schepsis AA. The role of arthroscopy in the assessment and treatment of tibial plateau fractures. Arthroscopy 1993; 9(5): 584-90.
[http://dx.doi.org/10.1016/S0749-8063(05)80410-4] [PMID: 8280333]

[64] Guanche CA, Markman AW. Arthroscopic management of tibial plateau fractures. Arthroscopy 1993; 9(4): 467-71.
[http://dx.doi.org/10.1016/S0749-8063(05)80324-X] [PMID: 8216581]

[65] Koechlin P, Nael JF, Bonnet JC, D?(tm)Ythurbide B, Apoil A. [Ligamentous lesions associated with fractures of the tibial plateau]. Acta Orthop Belg 1983; 49(6): 751-60.
[PMID: 6666577]

[66] Wilppula E, Bakalim G. Ligamentous tear concomitant with tibial condylar fracture. Acta Orthop Scand 1972; 43(4): 292-300.
[http://dx.doi.org/10.3109/17453677208991267] [PMID: 4651050]

[67] Bennett WF, Browner B. Tibial plateau fractures: a study of associated soft tissue injuries. J Orthop Trauma 1994; 8(3): 183-8.
[http://dx.doi.org/10.1097/00005131-199406000-00001] [PMID: 8027885]

[68] Vangsness CT Jr, Ghaderi B, Hohl M, Moore TM. Arthroscopy of meniscal injuries with tibial plateau fractures. J Bone Joint Surg Br 1994; 76(3): 488-90.
[PMID: 8175862]

[69] De Boeck H, Opdecam P. Posteromedial tibial plateau fractures. Operative treatment by posterior approach. Clin Orthop Relat Res 1995; (320): 125-8.
[PMID: 7586815]

[70] Daniel D, Rice T. Valgus-varus stability in a hinged cast used for controlled mobilization of the knee. J Bone Joint Surg Am 1979; 61(1): 135-6.
[PMID: 759423]

[71] Duwelius PJ, Connolly JF. Closed reduction of tibial plateau fractures. A comparison of functional and roentgenographic end results. Clin Orthop Relat Res 1988; (230): 116-26.
[PMID: 3365884]

[72] Hohl M. Part I fractures of the proximal tibia and fibula. 1991.

[73] Hohl M. Articular fractures of the proximal tibia. In: Evarts CM, Ed. Surgery of the musculoskeletal system. New York: Churchill-Livingstone 1993; pp. 3471-97.

[74] Zhang CY, Tao ZL, Zhang Q, *et al.* [Staging treatment for complex tibial metaphyseal fractures with external fixator]. Zhongguo Gu Shang 2014; 27(5): 425-9.
[PMID: 25167677]

[75]   Dirschl DR, Del Gaizo D. Staged management of tibial plateau fractures. Am J Orthop 2007; 36(4) (Suppl.): 12-7.
[PMID: 17547353]

[76]   Drennan DB, Locher FG, Maylahn DJ. Fractures of the tibial plateau. Treatment by closed reduction and spica cast. J Bone Joint Surg Am 1979; 61(7): 989-95.
[PMID: 489663]

[77]   Segal D, Mallik AR, Wetzler MJ, Franchi AV, Whitelaw GP. Early weight bearing of lateral tibial plateau fractures. Clin Orthop Relat Res 1993; (294): 232-7.
[PMID: 8358921]

[78]   Salter RB, Simmonds DF, Malcolm BW, Rumble EJ, MacMichael D, Clements ND. The biological effect of continuous passive motion on the healing of full-thickness defects in articular cartilage. An experimental investigation in the rabbit. J Bone Joint Surg Am 1980; 62(8): 1232-51.
[PMID: 7440603]

[79]   Onderko LL, Rehman S. Treatment of articular fractures with continuous passive motion. Orthop Clin North Am 2013; 44(3): 345-356, ix.
[http://dx.doi.org/10.1016/j.ocl.2013.04.002] [PMID: 23827837]

[80]   Brown GA, Sprague BL. Cast brace treatment of plateau and bicondylar fractures of the proximal tibia. Clin Orthop Relat Res 1976; (119): 184-93.
[PMID: 954310]

[81]   Keating JF. Tibial plateau fractures in the older patient. Bull Hosp Jt Dis 1999; 58(1): 19-23.
[PMID: 10431630]

[82]   Luria S, Liebergall M, Elishoov O, Kandel L, Mattan Y. Osteoporotic tibial plateau fractures: an underestimated cause of knee pain in the elderly. Am J Orthop 2005; 34(4): 186-8.
[PMID: 15913173]

[83]   Canale ST. 2008.

[84]   Furman BD, Strand J, Hembree WC, Ward BD, Guilak F, Olson SA. Joint degeneration following closed intraarticular fracture in the mouse knee: a model of posttraumatic arthritis. J Orthop Res 2007; 25(5): 578-92.
[http://dx.doi.org/10.1002/jor.20331] [PMID: 17266145]

[85]   Ballard BL, Antonacci JM, Temple-Wong MM, *et al.* Effect of tibial plateau fracture on lubrication function and composition of synovial fluid. J Bone Joint Surg Am 2012; 94(10): e64.
[http://dx.doi.org/10.2106/JBJS.K.00046] [PMID: 22617930]

[86]   Blokker CP, Rorabeck CH, Bourne RB. Tibial plateau fractures. An analysis of the results of treatment in 60 patients. Clin Orthop Relat Res 1984; (182): 193-9.
[PMID: 6546361]

[87]   Rademakers MV, Kerkhoffs GM, Sierevelt IN, Raaymakers EL, Marti RK. Operative treatment of 109 tibial plateau fractures: five- to 27-year follow-up results. J Orthop Trauma 2007; 21(1): 5-10.
[http://dx.doi.org/10.1097/BOT.0b013e31802c5b51] [PMID: 17211262]

[88]   ArA,en A, LA,ken S, Heir S, *et al.* Articular cartilage lesions in 993 consecutive knee arthroscopies. Am J Sports Med 2004; 32(1): 211-5.

[http://dx.doi.org/10.1177/0363546503259345] [PMID: 14754746]

[89]   Curl WW, Krome J, Gordon ES, Rushing J, Smith BP, Poehling GG. Cartilage injuries: a review of 31,516 knee arthroscopies. Arthroscopy 1997; 13(4): 456-60.
[http://dx.doi.org/10.1016/S0749-8063(97)90124-9] [PMID: 9276052]

[90]   Hjelle K, Solheim E, Strand T, Muri R, Brittberg M. Articular cartilage defects in 1,000 knee arthroscopies. Arthroscopy 2002; 18(7): 730-4.
[http://dx.doi.org/10.1053/jars.2002.32839] [PMID: 12209430]

[91]   Farmer JM, Martin DF, Boles CA, Curl WW. Chondral and osteochondral injuries. Diagnosis and management. Clin Sports Med 2001; 20(2): 299-320.
[http://dx.doi.org/10.1016/S0278-5919(05)70308-2] [PMID: 11398360]

[92]   Makino A, Muscolo DL, Puigdevall M, Costa-Paz M, Ayerza M. Arthroscopic fixation of osteochondritis dissecans of the knee: clinical, magnetic resonance imaging, and arthroscopic follow-up. Am J Sports Med 2005; 33(10): 1499-504.
[http://dx.doi.org/10.1177/0363546505274717] [PMID: 16009988]

[93]   Cain EL, Clancy WG. Treatment algorithm for osteochondral injuries of the knee. Clin Sports Med 2001; 20:321. Rev Med Devices 2006; 3: 585.

[94]   Frattini M, Vaienti E, Soncini G, Pogliacomi F. Tibial plateau fractures in elderly patients. Chir Organi Mov 2009; 93(3): 109-14.
[PMID: 19876712]

[95]   Mithoefer K, Williams RJ III, Warren RF, *et al.* The microfracture technique for the treatment of articular cartilage lesions in the knee. A prospective cohort study. J Bone Joint Surg Am 2005; 87(9): 1911-20.
[http://dx.doi.org/10.2106/JBJS.D.02846] [PMID: 16140804]

[96]   Gobbi A, Nunag P, Malinowski K. Treatment of full thickness chondral lesions of the knee with microfracture in a group of athletes. Knee Surg Sports Traumatol Arthrosc 2005; 13(3): 213-21.
[http://dx.doi.org/10.1007/s00167-004-0499-3] [PMID: 15146311]

[97]   Sankhala S S, Gupta S P, Sharma J C, Agarwal S. Tibial condylar fractures treated with traction and early mobilization (report on study of 75 cases). J Indian med Assosc 1990; 88(11): 11-309.

[98]   Bartha L, Vajda A, Duska Z, Rahmeh H, Hangody L. Autologous osteochondral mosaicplasty grafting. J Orthop Sports Phys Ther 2006; 36(10): 739-50.
[http://dx.doi.org/10.2519/jospt.2006.2182] [PMID: 17063836]

[99]   Chow JC, Hantes ME, Houle JB, Zalavras CG. Arthroscopic autogenous osteochondral transplantation for treating knee cartilage defects: a 2- to 5-year follow-up study. Arthroscopy 2004; 20(7): 681-90.
[http://dx.doi.org/10.1016/S0749-8063(04)00590-0] [PMID: 15346108]

[100] Convery FR, Akeson WH, Meyers MH. The operative technique of fresh osteochondral allografting of the knee. Oper Tech Orthop 1997; 7: 340.
[http://dx.doi.org/10.1016/S1048-6666(97)80038-9]

[101] Ghazavi MT, Pritzker KP, Davis AM, Gross AE. Fresh osteochondral allografts for post-traumatic osteochondral defects of the knee. J Bone Joint Surg Br 1997; 79(6): 1008-13.
[http://dx.doi.org/10.1302/0301-620X.79B6.7534] [PMID: 9393922]

[102] Gudas R, Kalesinskas RJ, Kimtys V, *et al.* A prospective randomized clinical study of mosaic osteochondral autologous transplantation versus microfracture for the treatment of osteochondral defects in the knee joint in young athletes. Arthroscopy 2005; 21(9): 1066-75.
[http://dx.doi.org/10.1016/j.arthro.2005.06.018] [PMID: 16171631]

[103] Jakob RP, Franz T, Gautier E, Mainil-Varlet P. Autologous osteochondral grafting in the knee: indication, results, and reflections. Clin Orthop Relat Res 2002; (401): 170-84.
[http://dx.doi.org/10.1097/00003086-200208000-00020] [PMID: 12151894]

[104] Karataglis D, Green MA, Learmonth DJ. Autologous osteochondral transplantation for the treatment of chondral defects of the knee. Knee 2006; 13(1): 32-5.
[http://dx.doi.org/10.1016/j.knee.2005.05.006] [PMID: 16125942]

[105] Ma HL, Hung SC, Wang ST, Chang MC, Chen TH. Osteochondral autografts transfer for post-traumatic osteochondral defect of the knee-2 to 5 years follow-up. Injury 2004; 35(12): 1286-92.
[http://dx.doi.org/10.1016/j.injury.2004.02.013] [PMID: 15561119]

[106] Szerb I, Hangody L, Duska Z, Kaposi NP. Mosaicplasty: long-term follow-up. Bull Hosp Jt Dis 2005; 63(1-2): 54-62.
[PMID: 16536220]

[107] Williams RJ III, Dreese JC, Chen CT. Chondrocyte survival and material properties of hypothermically stored cartilage: an evaluation of tissue used for osteochondral allograft transplantation. Am J Sports Med 2004; 32(1): 132-9.
[http://dx.doi.org/10.1177/0095399703258733] [PMID: 14754736]

[108] Shasha N, Krywulak S, Backstein D, Pressman A, Gross AE. Long-term follow-up of fresh tibial osteochondral allografts for failed tibial plateau fractures. J Bone Joint Surg Am 2003; 85-A (Suppl. 2): 33-9.
[PMID: 12721343]

[109] Rose T, Lill H, Hepp P, Josten C. Autologous osteochondral mosaicplasty for treatment of a posttraumatic defect of the lateral tibial plateau: a case report with two-year follow-up. J Orthop Trauma 2005; 19(3): 217-22.
[http://dx.doi.org/10.1097/00005131-200503000-00012] [PMID: 15758678]

[110] Matsusue Y, Kotake T, Nakagawa Y, Nakamura T. Arthroscopic osteochondral autograft transplantation for chondral lesion of the tibial plateau of the knee. Arthroscopy 2001; 17(6): 653-9.
[http://dx.doi.org/10.1053/jars.2001.22400] [PMID: 11447556]

[111] Wilson WJ, Jacobs JE. Patellar graft for severely depressed comminuted fractures of the lateral tibial condyle. J Bone Joint Surg Am 1952; 34-A(2): 436-42.
[http://dx.doi.org/10.1016/0002-9610(52)90010-X] [PMID: 14917712]

[112] Russell TA, Kumar A, Davidson RL, Klinar DF, Kuester DJ. Fibular head autograft. A salvage technique for severely comminuted lateral fractures of the tibial plateau: report of five cases. Am J Orthop 1996; 25(11): 766-71.
[PMID: 8959257]

[113] Bartlett W, Skinner JA, Gooding CR, *et al.* Autologous chondrocyte implantation *versus* matrix-induced autologous chondrocyte implantation for osteochondral defects of the knee: a prospective,

randomized study. J Bone Joint Surg 2005; 87B: 640.
[http://dx.doi.org/10.1302/0301-620X.87B5.15905]

[114] Behrens P, Bitter T, Kurz B, Russlies M. Matrix-associated autologous chondrocyte transplantation/implantation (MACT/MACI)--5-year follow-up. Knee 2006; 13(3): 194-202.
[http://dx.doi.org/10.1016/j.knee.2006.02.012] [PMID: 16632362]

[115] Bentley G, Biant LC, Carrington RW, *et al.* A prospective, randomized comparison of autologous chondrocyte implantation *versus* mosaicplasty for osteochondral defects in the knee. J Bone Joint Surg 2003; 85B: 223.
[http://dx.doi.org/10.1302/0301-620X.85B2.13543]

[116] Browne JE, Anderson AF, Arciero R, *et al.* Clinical outcome of autologous chondrocyte implantation at 5 years in US subjects. Clin Orthop Relat Res 2005; (436): 237-45.
[http://dx.doi.org/10.1097/00003086-200507000-00036] [PMID: 15995447]

[117] Fu FH, Zurakowski D, Browne JE, *et al.* Autologous chondrocyte implantation *versus* debridement for treatment of full-thickness chondral defects of the knee: an observational cohort study with 3-year follow-up. Am J Sports Med 2005; 33(11): 1658-66.
[http://dx.doi.org/10.1177/0363546505275148] [PMID: 16093543]

[118] Gillogly SD, Myers TH, Reinold MM. Treatment of full-thickness chondral defects in the knee with autologous chondrocyte implantation. J Orthop Sports Phys Ther 2006; 36(10): 751-64.
[http://dx.doi.org/10.2519/jospt.2006.2409] [PMID: 17063837]

[119] Gooding CR, Bartlett W, Bentley G, Skinner JA, Carrington R, Flanagan A. A prospective, randomised study comparing two techniques of autologous chondrocyte implantation for osteochondral defects in the knee: Periosteum covered versus type I/III collagen covered. Knee 2006; 13(3): 203-10.
[http://dx.doi.org/10.1016/j.knee.2006.02.011] [PMID: 16644224]

[120] HAä uselmann HJ. Healing enhancement with chondrocyte transplantation and other means. Sports Med Arthrosc Rev 1998; 6: 60.

[121] Henderson I, Gui J, Lavigne P. Autologous chondrocyte implantation: natural history of postimplantation periosteal hypertrophy and effects of repair-site debridement on outcome. Arthroscopy 2006; 22(12): 1318-1324.e1.
[http://dx.doi.org/10.1016/j.arthro.2006.07.057] [PMID: 17157731]

[122] Horas U, Pelinkovic D, Herr G, Aigner T, Schnettler R. Autologous chondrocyte implantation and osteochondral cylinder transplantation in cartilage repair of the knee joint. A prospective, comparative trial. J Bone Joint Surg Am 2003; 85-A(2): 185-92.
[PMID: 12571292]

[123] Minas T, Chiu R. Autologous chondrocyte implantation. Am J Knee Surg 2000; 13(1): 41-50.
[PMID: 11826924]

[124] Peterson L, Minas T, Brittberg M, Lindahl A. Treatment of osteochondritis dissecans of the knee with autologous chondrocyte transplantation: results at two to ten years. J Bone Joint Surg Am 2003; 85-A (Suppl. 2): 17-24.
[PMID: 12721341]

[125] Minas T, Peterson L. Chondrocyte transplantation. Oper Tech Orthop 1997; 7: 323.
[http://dx.doi.org/10.1016/S1048-6666(97)80036-5]

[126] Minas T, Peterson L. Advanced techniques in autologous chondrocyte transplantation. Clin Sports Med 1999; 18(1): 13-44, v-vi.
[http://dx.doi.org/10.1016/S0278-5919(05)70128-9] [PMID: 10028115]

[127] O?(tm)Driscoll SW. Technical considerations in periosteal grafting for osteochondral injuries. Clin Sports Med 2001; 20(2): 379-402, vii.
[http://dx.doi.org/10.1016/S0278-5919(05)70312-4] [PMID: 11398364]

[128] Robertson WB, Fick D, Wood DJ, Linklater JM, Zheng MH, Ackland TR. MRI and clinical evaluation of collagen-covered autologous chondrocyte implantation (CACI) at two years. Knee 2007; 14(2): 117-27.
[http://dx.doi.org/10.1016/j.knee.2006.11.009] [PMID: 17257849]

[129] Krishnan SP, Skinner JA, Carrington RW, Flanagan AM, Briggs TW, Bentley G. Collagen-covered autologous chondrocyte implantation for osteochondritis dissecans of the knee: two- to seven-year results. J Bone Joint Surg Br 2006; 88(2): 203-5.
[http://dx.doi.org/10.1302/0301-620X.88B2.17009] [PMID: 16434524]

[130] Gobbi A, Kon E, Berruto M, Francisco R, Filardo G, Marcacci M. Patellofemoral full-thickness chondral defects treated with Hyalograft-C: a clinical, arthroscopic, and histologic review. Am J Sports Med 2006; 34(11): 1763-73.
[http://dx.doi.org/10.1177/0363546506288853] [PMID: 16832129]

CHAPTER 5

Knee Arthroscopy and Tibial Plateau Fractures

Alessandro Aprato[1,*], Matheus Azi[2], Matteo Giachino[3] and Alessandro Massè[1]

[1] *University of Turin, Unit of Orthopaedics and Traumatology, Hospital San Luigi Gonzaga, Orbassano (Turin), Italy*

[2] *Manoel Victorino Hospital, Salvador, Brasil*

[3] *School of Orthopaedics and Traumatology, University of Turin (Turin), Italy*

Abstract: Arthroscopic-assisted fluoroscopic treatment of tibial plateau fractures has gained popularity in the last decade and is now indicated as one of the treatments of choice in Schatzker types 1, 2 and 3 fractures; it ensures optimal reduction and a stable fixation with plate or cannulated screws may be performed after reduction. In selected type 4 fractures arthroscopy may allow an evaluation of articular fracture reduction, thereby obviating the need for extensive arthrotomy. This chapter aims to review the technical points that are useful to the successful video-assisted management of tibial plateau fractures.

Keywords: Internal fixation, Knee arthroscopy, Tibial plateau fractures.

BACKGROUND

Arthroscopic-assisted fluoroscopic treatment is a minimally invasive alternative to standard open surgical techniques for tibial plateau fractures [1, 2]. The possible advantages are less postoperative swelling than open techniques and reduction of pain, risk of complications and recovery times. Several fractures patterns may be treated with this techniques but a rigorous indication should be respected.

---

* **Correspondence author Alessandro Aprato:** University of Turin, Unit of Orthopaedics and Traumatology, Hospital San Luigi Gonzaga, Regione Gonzole 10, 10043 - Orbassano (Turin), Italy; Tel: +390119026626; E-mail: ale_aprato@hotmail.com.

INDICATIONS

Many classification systems have been developed for proximal tibial fractures but the classification system proposed by Schatzker is the most widely used nowadays [3]. Its success relies on its clinical viability, it considers two fundamental lesions: cleavage and depression, along with their possible combinations. According to the Schatzker classification fractures type 1 (lateral split), type 2 (lateral split with depression) and type 3 (pure depression of the lateral plateau) are good indications for arthroscopic-assisted fluoroscopic treatment (Fig. **1**), In selected type 4 (medial plateau fracture with or without an intercondylar fracture) this technique may be used but invasive internal fixation erases several of the benefits from arthroscopic treatment, making percutaneous fixation a more reasonable choice in this type of fracture when treated with the arthroscopic method. However, extensive fixation may be warranted in the event of a comminuted fracture and in patients with osteoporosis. In type 5 (bicondylar fracture) and type 6 (unicondylar or bicondylar tibial plateau fracture with an extension that separates the metaphysis from the diaphysis) arthroscopy does not add advantages in respect to common open reduction and internal fixation.

BENEFIT AND RISKS

Arthroscopic-assisted fluoroscopic treatment presents many benefits: it allows to irrigate the joint, to remove loose bodies and/or free fragment and to treat associated soft tissue lesions. Associated meniscal tears is frequent in those cases, in literature its incidence varies from 2% to 47% [4, 5] and (in selected cases) meniscal suturing may be (indicated) appropriate whenever achievable, due to the reported high healing rate and the osteoarthritis risk intrinsically associated with the injury [6]. Lesions of the collateral ligaments is less common but should be sought routinely, as they may compromise knee stability and sometimes require surgical repair during the fracture fixation procedure. Damage to the anterior cruciate ligament (ACL) is common and reported in 4% to 32% of the cases [7, 8]. Schatzker types 4 and 6 fractures are more likely to have a ACL associated lesion [9]; it is generally preferred to treat bony avulsion at the same time as the tibial plateau, while midsubstance injury requires a second stage reconstruction, if indicated [10, 11]. Posterior cruciate ligament (PCL) lesions are less common.

Direct vision of the reduction and the chance of clinically testing the stability of the fracture are the most important advantages of this technique.

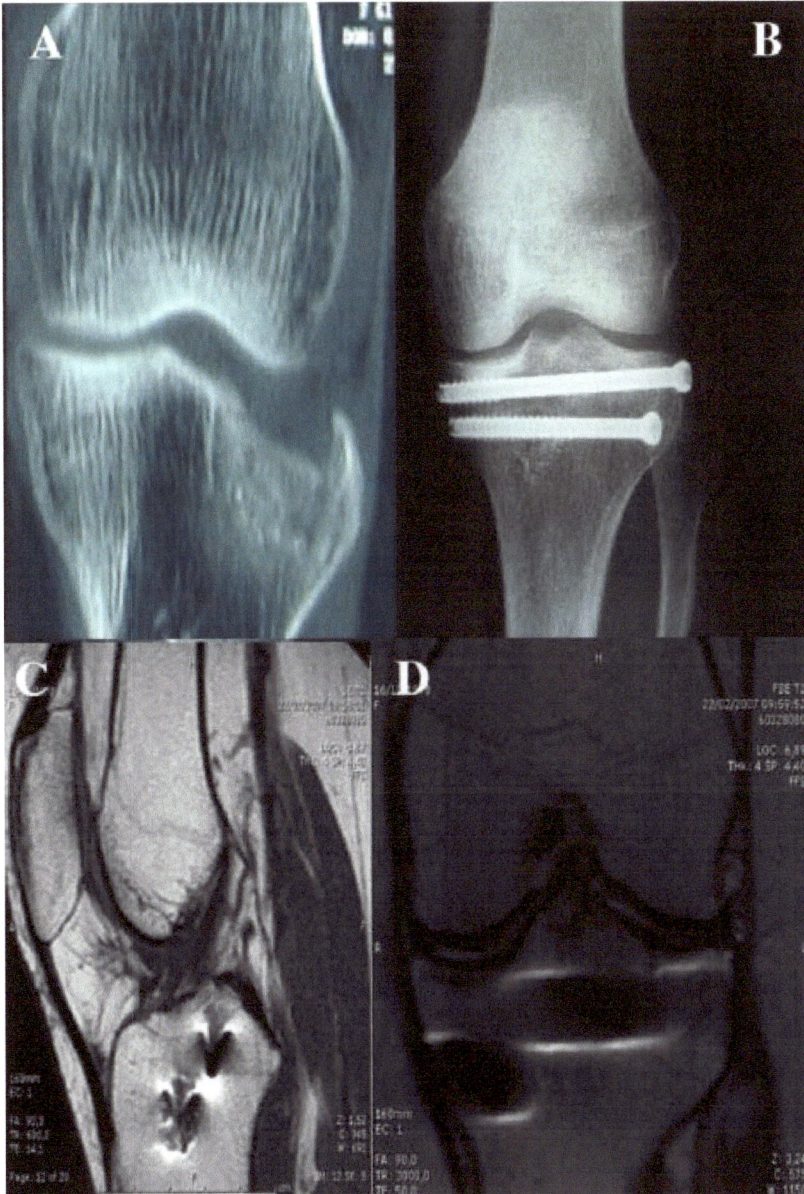

Fig. (1). Preoperative CT scan (**A**), post-operative X-rays (**B**) and MRI (**C** and **D**) images of a Schatzker type III fracture treated with arthroscopic assisted reduction and internal fixation [courtesy of dr. Francesco Atzori, San Luigi Hospital of Orbassano, Italy]).

Reduced risk of infection and reduced post-postoperative pain are related to minimal dissection of soft tissues [12, 13]. Risk of this procedure may be related to a poor intra-articular vision subsequent to excessive intra-articular bleeding, this may lead to iatrogenic injury or damage to the cartilage, ligaments, meniscus and even blood vessels or nerves.

Compartment syndrome due to fluid extravasation is the most dreaded complication but is also rare if gravity inflow used. A limited tourniquet time is also recommended to minimize this risk [29]. The pressure of the calf should be monitored during the procedure to minimize this risk [10].

SURGICAL TECHNIQUE

Surgical technique may be divided in 5 steps:

A. Patient position and clinical exam
B. Arthroscopic joint examination
C. Fracture reduction
D. Fracture fixation
E. Defect filling and wound closure

Patient Position and Clinical Exam

The patient is placed in supine position with a support or stirrup at the root of the limb so that limb mobility is unrestricted. Varus or valgus position may be required during reduction. A tourniquet may be used and placed as proximal as possible in the thigh.

Sterile access to the iliac crest should be prepared if an autologous graft has been planned. A high quality image amplifier should be used and its optimal position should be determined before draping: anteroposterior and lateral view should be easily performed during surgery. After anesthesia anteroposterior knee stability should be carefully but evaluated avoiding additional fracture displacement.

Arthroscopic Joint Examination

Conventional anterolateral and anteromedial portals are created and irrigation of the knee with saline is performed to achieve a good vision of the tibial plateau. The use of a pump has been criticized but facilitate joint lavage, provided pressure is no higher than 50 mmHg.

If evacuation of the hematoma is challenging, a third portal may be created in a superolateral position and used for a cannula to help hematoma evacuation.

When intra-articular visibility becomes sufficient, a shaver can be introduced to remove the clots and loose bodies.

A 360 degrees evaluation should be performed to identify the bone and cartilage lesions, as well as any damage to other structures such as the menisci and ligaments. Associated lesions have prognostic significance and may require additional surgical procedures in future. Fractures that are very near the periphery of the plateau and partly located under the meniscus may be difficult to visualize. In those cases, a suture wire may useful to retract the meniscus [14].

Fracture Reduction

Reduction is commonly easy to achieve in Schatzker type 1 fracture with traction and varus stress of the joint. Fluoroscopic guidance may be useful if arthroscopic vision is suboptimal. If reduction is not sufficient, a fragment may be elevated to the level of the joint surface with a lever or a ball-joint forceps.

Reduction may also be achieved inserting one or two K-wires into the lateral plateau using them as a joystick to elevate the fragment and to correct any rotational displacement. When fracture reduction remains impossible, bone fragments should be dis-impacted with a slender spatula or palpation hook slipped into the fracture site [14].

Fluoroscopic guidance of instruments should be used to avoid worsening the bone lesions.

When the fragment is in the ideal position, temporary fixation is achieved with K-wires. Those wires should ideally be placed parallel to the joint surface and about 1 cm under the joint surface in order to be used also for subsequent fixation.

In Schatzker type 3 fractures (isolated depression) the impacted fragment height should be restored. It may be achieved as described before or through the metaphysis. A small skin incision on the lateral or medial metaphysis may be done and the bone exposed. A 2*2 cm square of cortex is removed and a bone plunger introduced. The plunger advancement toward the depression zone is monitored under fluoroscopic guidance in both 2 views and it should stop about 2 cm under the depressed area.

At this point, the fragment could be elevated with a bone impactor by applying force with a small hammer so as to obtain a satisfactory reduction. The key to good-quality reduction of the depressed joint surface is application of the elevating force at the center of the depression.

Faultless technique is required to avoid worsening the displacement or penetrating into the joint cavity through the joint surface. If force is not applied nearly perpendicular to the joint surface, iatrogenic lesion may be more frequent.

Slight overcorrection of the joint surface depression followed by flexion of the knee is desirable to allow the femoral condyle to shape the joint surface. Temporary stabilization is then performed as previously described.

In Schatzker type 2 fractures the previously described technical stratagems should be used in combination. In selected Schatzker type 4 those technique may be helpful to partially reduce the most lateral fragments but in most of the cases an open reduction should be performed.

Fracture Fixation

Although some authors advocate the use of a plate in those cases, lateral tibial plateau fractures may be fixed using two or three large-diameter (6.5 mm) cannulated screws (Fig. **1**).

They are commonly inserted percutaneously, in combination with a washer. Care should be taken to avoid excessive screws tightening, which can adversely affect reduction quality. As mentioned above there is no consensus on whether to prefer screw or plate fixation, both biomechanical and cadaver studies didn't manage to give an unequivocal response, although many authors have proved clinical reliability of screws[3, 15 - 18]. In Schatzker type 4 fractures, cannulated screws may not be sufficient to fix the fractures [19].

Defect Filling and Wound Closure

There is no consensus about defect filling but literature shows that main risk factor for secondary displacement is a large bony defect under the depression. Although a symposium (1999 SOFCOT symposium, Société Française de Chirurgie Orthopédique et Traumatologique) found no significant difference between patients managed with and without bone grafting, filling seems a good option if the depression is greater than 6 mm or patients present poor bone quality [20 - 23].

Defect may be filled with autologous iliac crest, frozen allogeneic bone grafts, freeze-dried allogeneic bone or synthetic bone substitutes [24 - 27]. Pros and contras of those materials are well known to the orthopaedic surgeons.

After defect filling, final check of articular surface is arthroscopically made and wound closure may be performed.

POST-OPERATIVE CARE

Drainage may be used according to surgeon habits.

Mobilization might start after 24 hours or as soon as possible and continue passive motion may be helpful in the post-operative period. Weight-bearing is allowed only 8 to 10 weeks after surgery. Thromboembolism prophylaxis is given until the resumption of weight-bearing.

RESULTS

The majority of the studies agree that arthroscopic-assisted fluoroscopic treatment is an effective and safe procedure, although a definitive consensus on whether to prefer the latter to the standard open surgical techniques has yet to be found.

Post-operative clinical and radiological assessments have been carried out by a considerable number of authors, along with the evaluation of osteoarthritic evolution and further complications. However, two recent systematic reviews were published to summarize the last fifteen years of literature on the topic, bringing a clear overview of the technique outcome at a mean follow up of 52,4 months [28, 29].

Clinical outcome can be evaluated with common scales including the Rasmussen scoring system, which is one of the most widespread and specifically focused on tibial plateau; the radiologic counterpart of the scale is also validated for radiographic appraisal [30]. The overall clinical score reported a 90.5% of the patients facing good/excellent results, with a 90.9% of them satisfied after procedure [29]. it is remarkable that one study outlined an 89% of good or excellent clinical outcome considering only Schatzker type V or VI fractures [13]. In the sportsmen sub-group Scheerlinck *et al.* and Holzach *et al.* observed a return to the previous activity level respectively in 63% and 87% [4, 31]. Even in the cases of tibial plateau fracture with posterior commitment (present in 10 to 15% of Schatzker type 1 and 2 fractures, and in 22 to 76% of Schatzker type 4 to 6 [32]) the use of the arthroscopic-assisted reduction in the treatment of 25 cases with postero-medial involvement lead to 92% of good or excellent clinical and radiological results [33].

The radiological outcome after treatment was found to be good or excellent, according to the radiologic Rasmussen scoring system, in at least 63% of the patients in each case series [28].

The onset of secondary osteoarthritis is the most inconstant data emerging from the records; systematic reviews attest its incidence between 0% and 63%. This significant discrepancy is due to a multitude of factors that influence osteoarthritis development, including age of the patient, alignment of the lower limb, meniscus integrity and articular step-offs; previous arthritic cartilage lesions is also believed to negatively affect the clinical outcome after intervention [13, 23, 34, 35]. A significant narrowing of the joint space, however, became visible after more than 3 years of follow up in 10% to 30% of patients [4, 7, 31].

Dreadful complications like compartment syndrome, deep infection and deep venous thrombosis have to be considered rare circumstances [15, 18, 35] and no life-threatening situations have been recorded. In a meta-analysis involving 610 knees treated with the method only 6 severe complications were reported with 1 case of compartment syndrome and no amputations [29].

CONCLUSION

In conclusion the arthroscopic-assisted fluoroscopic treatment is an important method to assist the reduction of tibial plateau fractures. Despite its benefits, especially in reducing the surgical aggression to the soft tissue, its should be used without compromising the principles of treatment of articular fractures of anatomic reduction with absolute stability allowing early and safe mobilization.

CONFLICT OF INTEREST

The author confirms that author has no conflict of interest to declare for this publication.

ACKNOWLEDGEMENTS

Declared none.

REFERENCES

[1]   Caspari RB, Hutton PM, Whipple TL, Meyers JF. The role of arthroscopy in the management of tibial plateau fractures. Arthroscopy 1985; 1(2): 76-82.
[http://dx.doi.org/10.1016/S0749-8063(85)80035-9] [PMID: 4091921]

[2]   Jennings JE. Arthroscopic management of tibial plateau fractures. Arthroscopy 1985; 1(3): 160-8.
[http://dx.doi.org/10.1016/S0749-8063(85)80003-7] [PMID: 4096767]

[3]   Schatzker J, McBroom R, Bruce D. The tibial plateau fracture. The Toronto experience 1968--1975. Clin Orthop Relat Res 1979; (138): 94-104.
[PMID: 445923]

[4]   Holzach P, Matter P, Minter J. Arthroscopically assisted treatment of lateral tibial plateau fractures in skiers: use of a cannulated reduction system. J Orthop Trauma 1994; 8(4): 273-81.
[http://dx.doi.org/10.1097/00005131-199408000-00001] [PMID: 7965287]

[5]   Vangsness CT Jr, Ghaderi B, Hohl M, Moore TM. Arthroscopy of meniscal injuries with tibial plateau fractures. J Bone Joint Surg Br 1994; 76(3): 488-90.
[PMID: 8175862]

[6]   Ruiz-Ibán MÁ, Diaz-Heredia J, Elías-Martín E, Moros-Marco S, Cebreiro Martinez Del Val I. Repair of meniscal tears associated with tibial plateau fractures: a review of 15 cases. Am J Sports Med 2012; 40(10): 2289-95.
[http://dx.doi.org/10.1177/0363546512457552] [PMID: 22962298]

[7]   Cassard X, Beaufils P, Blin JL, Hardy P. [Osteosynthesis under arthroscopic control of separated tibial plateau fractures. 26 case reports]. Rev Chir Orthop Repar Appar Mot 1999; 85(3): 257-66. [In French].
        [PMID: 10422131]

[8]   Gill TJ, Moezzi DM, Oates KM, Sterett WI. Arthroscopic reduction and internal fixation of tibial plateau fractures in skiing. Clin Orthop Relat Res 2001; (383): 243-9.
        [http://dx.doi.org/10.1097/00003086-200102000-00028] [PMID: 11210961]

[9]   Abdel-Hamid MZ, Chang CH, Chan YS, *et al.* Arthroscopic evaluation of soft tissue injuries in tibial plateau fractures: retrospective analysis of 98 cases. Arthroscopy 2006; 22(6): 669-75.
        [http://dx.doi.org/10.1016/j.arthro.2006.01.018] [PMID: 16762707]

[10]   Burdin G. Arthroscopic management of tibial plateau fractures: surgical technique. Orthop Traumatol Surg Res 2013; 99(1) (Suppl.): S208-18.
        [http://dx.doi.org/10.1016/j.otsr.2012.11.011] [PMID: 23347755]

[11]   Rossi R, Bonasia DE, Blonna D, Assom M, Castoldi F. Prospective follow-up of a simple arthroscopic-assisted technique for lateral tibial plateau fractures: results at 5 years. Knee 2008; 15(5): 378-83.
        [http://dx.doi.org/10.1016/j.knee.2008.04.001] [PMID: 18571417]

[12]   Chan YS. Arthroscopy- assisted surgery for tibial plateau fractures. Chang Gung Med J 2011; 34(3): 239-47.
        [PMID: 21733353]

[13]   Chan YS, Yuan LJ, Hung SS, *et al.* Arthroscopic-assisted reduction with bilateral buttress plate fixation of complex tibial plateau fractures. Arthroscopy 2003; 19(9): 974-84.
        [http://dx.doi.org/10.1016/j.arthro.2003.09.038] [PMID: 14608317]

[14]   Perez Carro L. Arthroscopic management of tibial plateau fractures: special techniques. Arthroscopy 1997; 13(2): 265-7.
        [http://dx.doi.org/10.1016/S0749-8063(97)90168-7] [PMID: 9127091]

[15]   Denny LD, Keating EM, Engelhardt JA, Saha S. A comparison of fixation techniques in tibial plateau fractures. Orthop Trans 1984; 10: 388-9.

[16]   Koval KJ, Polatsch D, Kummer FJ, Cheng D, Zuckerman JD. Split fractures of the lateral tibial plateau: evaluation of three fixation methods. J Orthop Trauma 1996; 10(5): 304-8.
        [http://dx.doi.org/10.1097/00005131-199607000-00003] [PMID: 8814570]

[17]   Boisrenoult P, Bricteux S, Beaufils P, Hardy P. Vis *versus* plaque vissée dans les fractures séparationenfoncement du plateau tibial latéral. Rev Chir Orthop Repar Appar Mot 2000; 86: 707-11. [In French].

[18]   Patil S, Mahon A, Green S, McMurtry I, Port A. A biomechanical study comparing a raft of 3.5 mm cortical screws with 6.5 mm cancellous screws in depressed tibial plateau fractures. Knee 2006; 13(3): 231-5.
        [http://dx.doi.org/10.1016/j.knee.2006.03.003] [PMID: 16647262]

[19]   Cift H, Cetik O, Kalaycioglu B, Dirikoglu MH, Ozkan K, Eksioglu F. Biomechanical comparison of plate-screw and screw fixation in medial tibial plateau fractures (Schatzker 4). A model study. Orthop

Traumatol Surg Res 2010; 96(3): 263-7.
[http://dx.doi.org/10.1016/j.otsr.2009.11.016] [PMID: 20488145]

[20]   Chauvaux D, Le Huec JC. Arthroscopie et fracture du plateau tibial : faut-il combler ou non? Annalesde la Société franc̦aised'arthroscopie. Montpellier: Sauramps médical 1999; pp. 5-143. [In French]

[21]   Le Huec JC. Fractures articulaires récentes de l'extrémité supérieure du tibia de l'adulte Cahiers d'enseignement de la SOFCOT. Paris: Expansion Scientifique franc̦aise 1996; pp. 97-117. [In French]

[22]   Chauvaux D, Le Huec JC, Roger D, Le Rebeller A. Traitement chirurgical sous contrôle arthroscopique des fractures des plateaux tibiaux. Rev Chir Orthop Repar Appar Mot 1991; 77(1): 288. [In French].

[23]   Roerdink WH, Oskam J, Vierhout PA. Arthroscopically assisted osteosynthesis of tibial plateau fractures in patients older than 55 years. Arthroscopy 2001; 17(8): 826-31.
[http://dx.doi.org/10.1016/S0749-8063(01)90005-2] [PMID: 11600979]

[24]   Goulet JA, Senunas LE, DeSilva GL, Greenfield ML. Autogenous iliac crest bone graft. Complications and functional assessment. Clin Orthop Relat Res 1997; (339): 76-81.
[http://dx.doi.org/10.1097/00003086-199706000-00011] [PMID: 9186204]

[25]   Palmer SH, Gibbons CL, Athanasou NA. The pathology of bone allograft. J Bone Joint Surg Br 1999; 81(2): 333-5.
[http://dx.doi.org/10.1302/0301-620X.81B2.9320] [PMID: 10204946]

[26]   Lubowitz JH, Vance KJ, Ayala M, Guttmann D, Reid JB III. Interference screw technique for arthroscopic reduction and internal fixation of compression fractures of the tibial plateau. Arthroscopy 2006; 22(12): 1359.e1-3.
[http://dx.doi.org/10.1016/j.arthro.2006.04.110] [PMID: 17157737]

[27]   Frankenburg EP, Goldstein SA, Bauer TW, Harris SA, Poser RD. Biomechanical and histological evaluation of a calcium phosphate cement. J Bone Joint Surg Am 1998; 80(8): 1112-24.
[PMID: 9730120]

[28]   Chen HW, Liu GD, Wu LJ. Clinical and radiological outcomes following arthroscopic-assisted management of tibial plateau fractures: a systematic review. Knee Surg Sports Traumatol Arthrosc 2014. [Epub ahead of print].
[PMID: 25246171]

[29]   Chen XZ, Liu CG, Chen Y, Wang LQ, Zhu QZ, Lin P. Arthroscopy-Assisted Surgery for Tibial Plateau Fractures 2014.

[30]   Rasmussen PS. Impairment of knee joint stability as an indi- cation for surgical treatment. J Bone Joint Surg Am 1973; 55: 1331-50.
[PMID: 4586086]

[31]   Scheerlinck T, Ng CS, Handelberg F, Casteleyn PP. Medium-term results of percutaneous, arthroscopically-assisted osteosynthesis of fractures of the tibial plateau. J Bone Joint Surg Br 1998; 80(6): 959-64.
[http://dx.doi.org/10.1302/0301-620X.80B6.8687] [PMID: 9853485]

[32]   Yang G, Zhai Q, Zhu Y, Sun H, Putnis S, Luo C. The incidence of posterior tibial plateau fracture: an

investigation of 525 fractures by using a CT-based classification system. Arch Orthop Trauma Surg 2013; 133(7): 929-34.
[http://dx.doi.org/10.1007/s00402-013-1735-4] [PMID: 23589062]

[33]   Chiu C-H, Cheng C-Y, Tsai M-C, *et al.* Arthroscopy-assisted reduction of posteromedial tibial plateau fractures with buttress plate and cannulated screw construct. Arthroscopy 2013; 29(8): 1346-54.
[http://dx.doi.org/10.1016/j.arthro.2013.05.003] [PMID: 23820261]

[34]   Ohdera T, Tokunaga M, Hiroshima S, Yoshimoto E, Tokunaga J, Kobayashi A. Arthroscopic management of tibial plateau fractures--comparison with open reduction method. Arch Orthop Trauma Surg 2003; 123(9): 489-93.
[http://dx.doi.org/10.1007/s00402-003-0510-3] [PMID: 12720016]

[35]   Siegler J, Galissier B, Marcheix PS, Charissoux JL, Mabit C, Arnaud JP. Percutaneous fixation of tibial plateau fractures under arthroscopy: a medium term perspective. Orthop Traumatol Surg Res 2011; 97(1): 44-50.
[http://dx.doi.org/10.1016/j.otsr.2010.08.005] [PMID: 21233036]

[36]   Asik M, Cetik O, Talu U, Sozen YV. Arthroscopy-assisted operative management of tibial plateau fractures. Knee Surg Sports Traumatol Arthrosc 2002; 10(6): 364-70.
[http://dx.doi.org/10.1007/s00167-002-0310-2] [PMID: 12444516]

CHAPTER 6

Balloon Tibioplasty

Francesco Atzori[1,*] and **Davide Deledda**[2]

[1] *University of Turin, Unit of Orthopaedics and Traumatology, Hospital San Luigi Gonzaga, Orbassano (Turin), Italy*

[2] *School of Orthopaedics and Traumatology, University of Turin, (Turin), Italy*

Abstract: The target of tibial plateau fracture management is to obtain an anatomical reduction and an early knee mobilization. Balloon tibioplasty is a new minimally invasive technique adapted for reduction of depressed tibial plateau fracture and it represents a surgical method to restore the cartilage surface. The advantages of balloon tibioplasty are: minimally invasive technique and creation of symmetric space inside the proximal tibia bone that reduces stresses on the fracture. The bone gap above the tibia plateau is filled with ceramic bone cement through a small cortex bone window. It is a technique that requires a correct learning curve, but it may be a useful tool that makes the reduction of selected depressed tibial plateau fractures easier.

Keywords: Articular fractures, Balloon, Fixation, Osteoplasty, Tibial plateau, Tibioplasty.

INTRODUCTION

The tibial plateau fractures are intra-articular fractures and they are divided into high and low energy lesions. They are often associated with ligament injuries and secondary long-term complications are frequent (*e.g.* post-traumatic arthrosis and a valgus deformity). Nowadays surgeons pay more attention to soft tissues preservation [1]. Mini-invasive techniques have reduced long-term complications and they are able to preserve the normal functions of the knee [2, 3]. The main target of these techniques is to restore the articular surface the most anatomically

* **Correspondence author Francesco Atzori:** University of Turin, Unit of Orthopaedics and Traumatology, Hospital San Luigi Gonzaga, Regione Gonzole 10, 10043, Orbassano (Turin), Italy; Tel: +390119026626; E-mail: f_atz@libero.it.

as possible, preserving the stability and the load axis of the knee [4].

ETIOLOGY

The tibial plateau fractures are often due to a trauma with a direct axial load, more commonly in valgus stress position [5]. The femoral condyle transfers the load directly on the tibial plateau. Injury types are related to the position, the longitudinal axis and the flexion degree of knee. The lateral tibial plateau is more involved than the medial one and it is correlated to the axis of the knee (usually valgus) [6]. Many other factors influence the etiology of the lesion, such as the age [7, 8] and bone quality of the patients. Ligament and capsular injuries are commonly associated to bone fractures in younger, because of the cancellous bone is more resistant than that in elderly patients [9].

DIAGNOSIS

Radiographic evaluation involves standard AP and LL image. Additional oblique projection are useful to better determinate the fracture [10]. CT Scan with 3D reconstructions has increased the accuracy of diagnosis and the fracture tridimensional study [11]. Moreover MRI evaluates soft tissue associated injuries in a non-invasive way compared to arthroscopic study [12].

CLASSIFICATION

Many classification scores have been proposed. Currently the most widely used is the classification proposed by Schatzker. It is the first classification that divides medial and lateral plateau fractures. The I type is a lateral fracture with one bone fragment, the II type is a splinted fracture associated with depression of the plateau. The III type is a pure central depression, while condyles are intact. The IV type involves medial plateau and it is divided in to two subgroups: type A is a split-fracture and type B is a fracture with depression of the bone. The V type is an inverted "Y" fracture that involves both tibial condyles, without metaphysis or diaphysis fragments. The VI and last type is a complete fracture between metaphysis or diaphysis segments [13]. Other classifications commonly used are: the Hohl scoring system (the first that have been proposed), Moore and AO scoring system [14, 15].

BALLOON TIBIOPLASTY

The common fracture patterns encountered are split depression (OTA Type B3, Schatzker Type II) and lateral depression injuries (OTA type B2, Schatzker type III) in elderly patients, due to osteopenia or osteoporosis. The bone depression needs to be elevated through a surgical made bone window in the proximal tibia without opening the joint. The tibial plateau is covered by hyaline cartilage that can be damaged easily; every mini-invasive surgical approach may lead to an intra-articular penetration.

Pizanis *et al.* described a mini-invasive technique: he used an inflatable kyphoplasty balloon as a reduction aid. It allows to minimize the cortex bone window and increases the mechanical force needed to elevate the depression.

Pre-Operative Planning

A correct pre-operative planning is very useful to determinate the type and the deepness of the fracture. Standard AP and lateral radiographs should be associated with CT scan to determinate correctly the landmarks, which are the tibial spine and the head of the fibula. It is important to evaluate the cartilage surface and the posterior part of the lateral tibial plateau. Using standard fluoroscopic study (AP and lateral projections), the introducer should be placed between 2 to 10 mm below the deepest part of the fracture.

Surgical Technique

The patient is placed in supine position with the knee flexed at 45 degrees. The surgical skin incision is a limited exposure of the lateral proximal tibia. Arhtroscopy is useful to evaluate the articular surface; in case of difficult evaluation of the articular joint, a small transverse arthrotomy could be performed. Using minimally invasive techniques a fragment locking T-plate locked with cortical screws (Synthes, Freiburg, Germany) is placed on the antero-lateral surface of the proximal tibia as a lateral support. An assistant prepares the balloon (IBT) on the back table at the beginning of the surgery. The skin incision is performed on the medial side of the tibial plateau. The Osteo Introducer (Kyphon, Sunnyvale, CA) is composed of an external cannula, a spindle with an acute tip (Trocar). Using the radiographic landmarks made before, the surgeon could place the introducer; the cortex could be broken using a small hammer or a 3.2 diameter drill. The cannula has a 4 mm diameter and it is inserted below the fracture. The bone void device (Kyphon), filled with contrast solution, allows the surgeon to observe of the reduction of the fracture. In case of large tibial plateau depression more than one void filler devices can be used. The fluoroscopic images are important to estimate the correct reduction checking the line fracture. The contrast solution quantity is equal to cement quantity (HydroSetTM; Stryker, Portage, MI). The balloon could be removed and the cement is injected, the mean volume is about 4 to 6 mL. 12 to 15 minutes is the time required for the cement to polymerize and then the plate is locked with screws.

A complication that can occur is a secondary loss of reduction, after balloon deflation; Kirschner wires can be used temporally to keep the reduction while the cement polymerizes.

The figures summarize procedure steps:

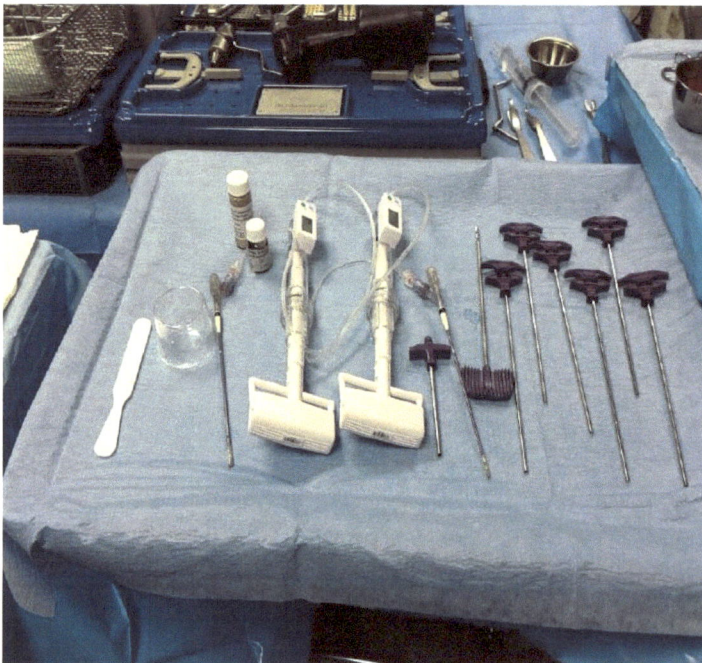

Fig. (1). Balloon tibioplasty tool.

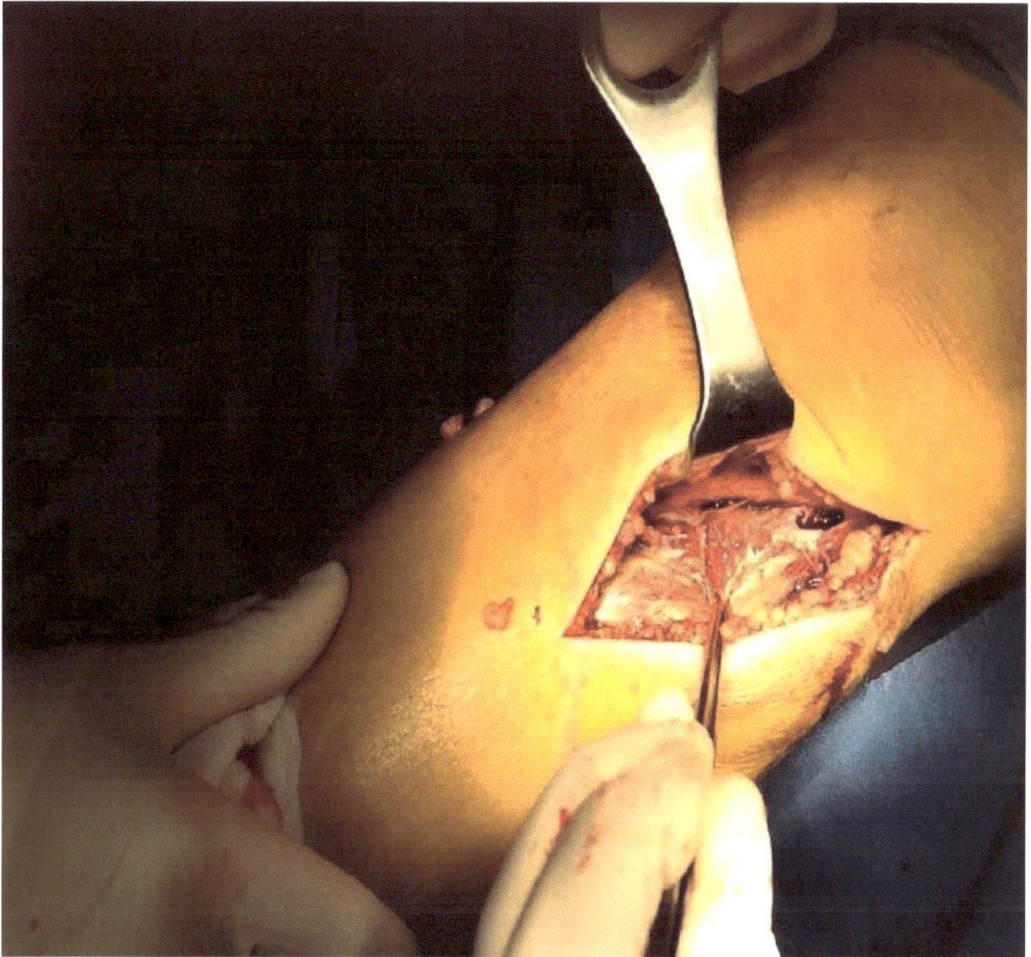

Fig. (2). Surgical exposure.

After Surgery Managements

A rehabilitation program is important after the surgery to achieve a rapid and complete functional restoration. Patients could mobilize the knee, without brace, according to the pain. For 4 weeks is completely avoiding weight bearing. Full weight bearing could be achieved gradually 6 weeks after surgery, using crunches. During this period, the thromboprophylaxis with heparin must be performed. A radiographic control every 30 days should be performed using standard X-ray, for 90 days after surgery.

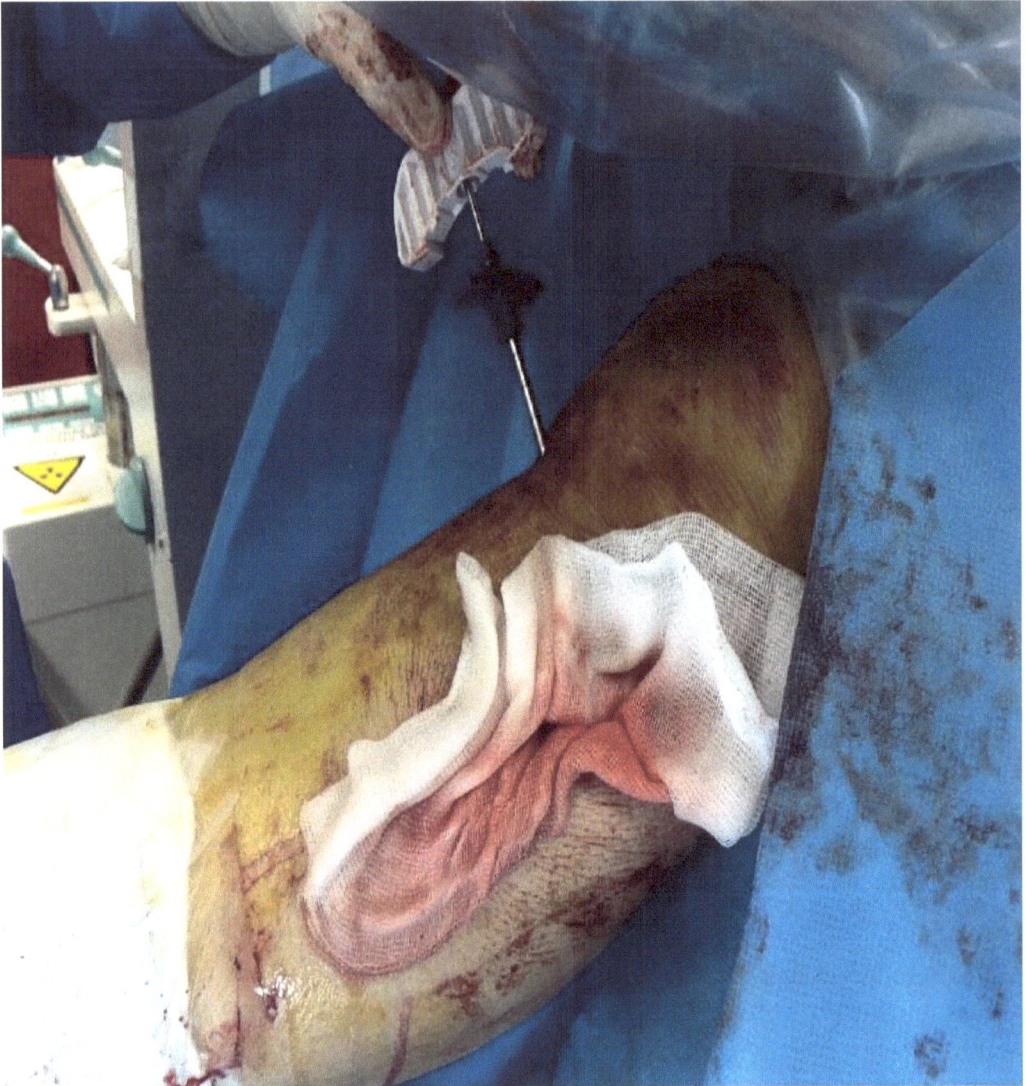

Fig. (3a). Bone void filler device under fluoroscopic images.

Literature Analysis

Tibial plateau fractures are very common, especially in elderly people. Many mini-invasive surgical techniques have been proposed; they demonstrated good clinical result with a complete restoration of knee function. The ballon tibioplasty is a brand new technique derived from the spine surgery. It is similar to vertebral osteoplasty: the bone vertebral soma shape can be restored and stabilized with cement using a insufflated balloon. The concept is the same. The depression of the tibial plateau can be treated with a balloon insufflated with a contrast solution, the cartilage surface is restored under radiographic control and then stabilized. This surgery is a mini invasive solution, that is suitable for elderly. It can prevent skin incision delayed repair, vascular diseases and reduces infection.

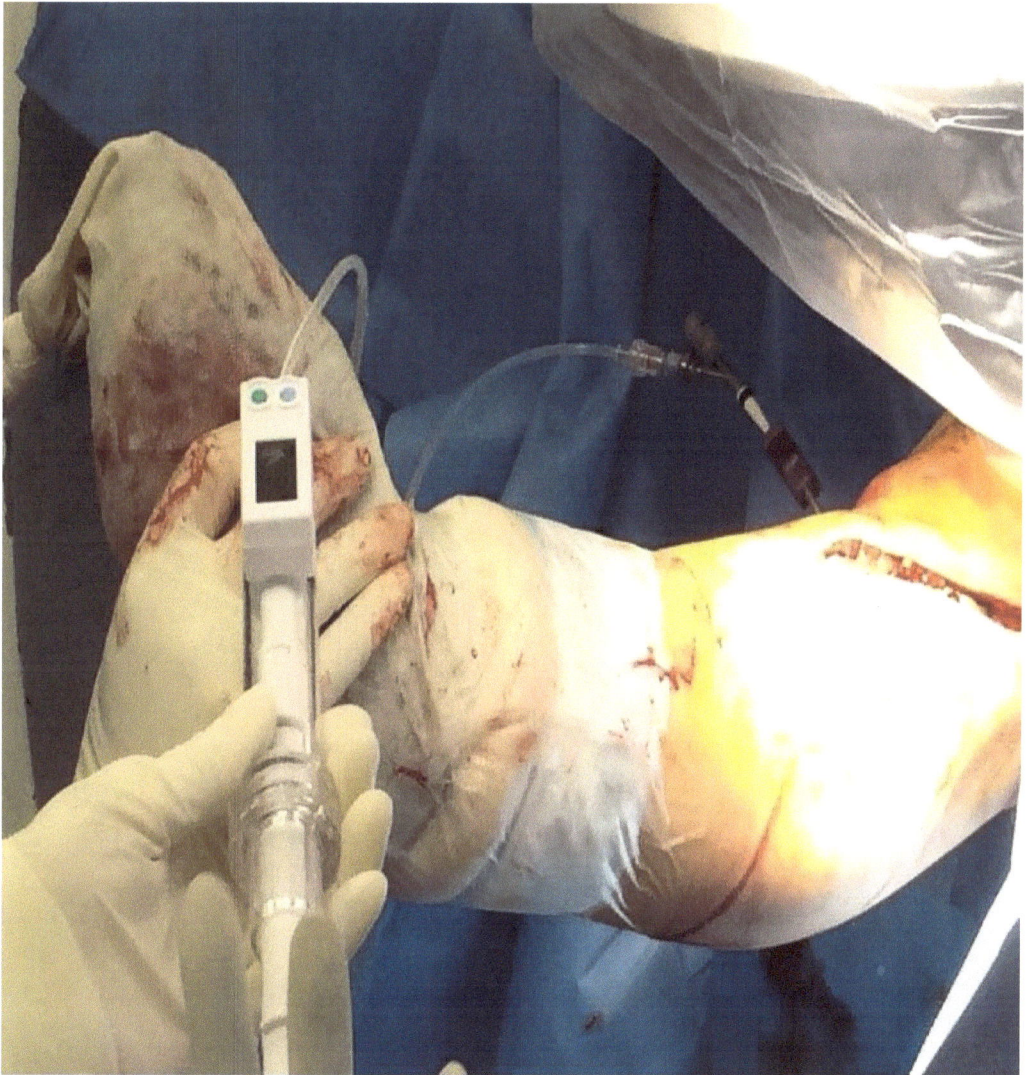

Fig. (3b). Bone void filler device under fluoroscopic images.

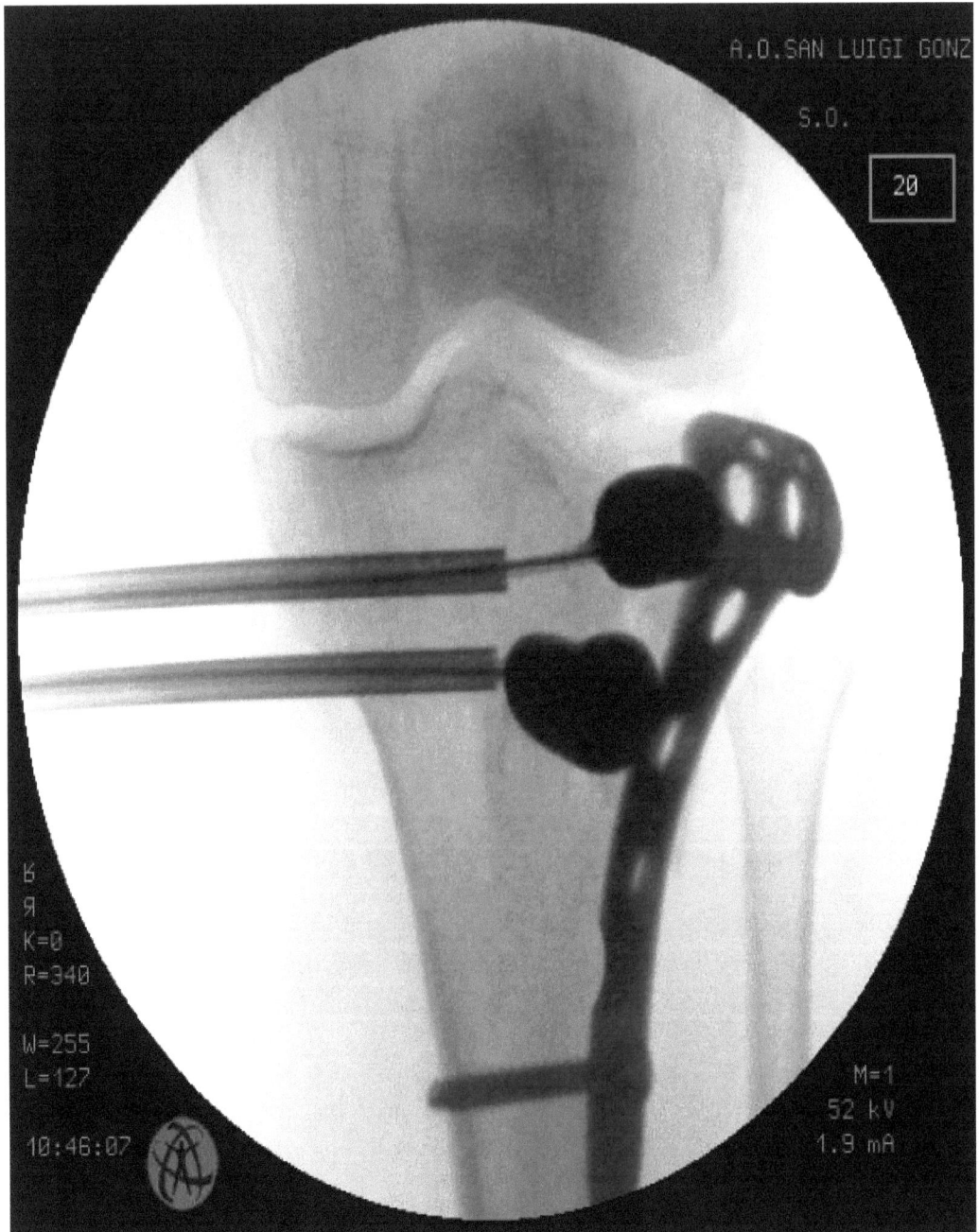

Fig. (4). Intraoperative fluoroscopic control.

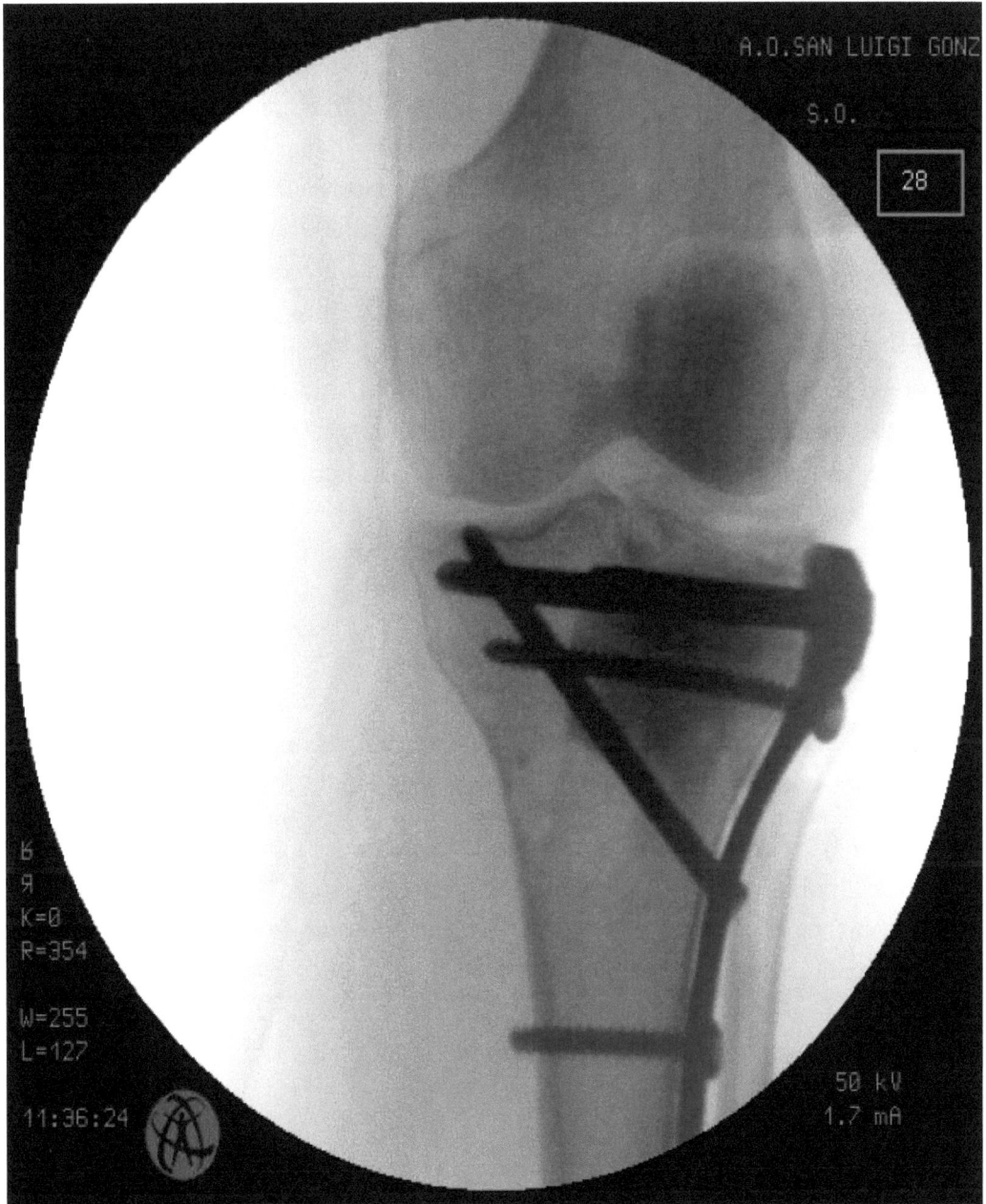

Fig. (5). Final result.

Pizanis *et al.* [16] described the balloon tibioplasty technique: between January 2007 and December 2010, 5 of 186 patients with displaced tibial plateau fractures were treated using balloon tibioplasty technique. Patients had a low-energy trauma with no soft tissue damage. They were either young adults or elderly, from 44 to 80 years. Four patients had a lateral depression fracture (Schatzker III) and 1 patient had a split depression fracture (Schatzker type II). The preoperative depression measured 8–12 mm on standard radiographs and CT scans. The timing of the surgery was 7–9 days after trauma. The reduction has been considered excellent at the time of the surgery, no cartilage damages were found, with no modifications after 8 weeks. The short term evaluation was from about 12 to 36 months: no complications or fracture dislocation were detected. Mobilization was performed from the first postoperative day and full range of motion was achieved before the discharge (6 days for young people to 22 for elderly). All patients expressed a complete satisfaction with the treatment at the last follow-up, concerning operative outcomes and functional recovery compared to activities performed before the injury. The functional evaluation was performed using the Rasmussen and Lysholm scores yielded, which results were 28 to 30 points (30 points maximum) before surgery and 95 to 100 points (100 points maximum) after surgery.

Other authors described the balloon tibioplasty, but no mid and long term result are available at the moment [17, 18].

Broome *et al.* described a balloon reduction technique for distal radius and proximal tibial fractures in cadavers [17]. Six proximal tibias (intra-articular depression-type fractures on the medial and lateral side) were treated using the inflatable balloon to reduce the depression. CT scan study allowed to measure the restoration of the normal anatomy. The balloon reduction system was equivalent to conventional methods of reduction at short term. It offers the advantage of being minimally invasive.

Ahrens *et al.* [19] described a new technique on cadaver available for clinical applications. He adapted the inflatable instruments of the kiphoplasty and used the balloon technique to reduce depressed fractures of the tibial plateau. The technique can be compared to a standard reduction concerning clinical and radiological outcomes, but it demonstrated advantages of a mini invasive technique and a low collateral damage (a described complication of minimally invasive procedures).

Jordan *et al*. described a study in 2014 [20] as single-centred randomised trial. 24 adult patients with both a depressed or split depressed tibial plateau fracture were divided in to the two treatment groups. They compared standard methods of reduction to the mini-invasive one. Reduction was the main target. They evaluated any surgical complication and also patient satisfaction. Principal analysis was the success of fracture reduction comparing different methods.

CONCLUSION

Tibial plateau fractures occur commonly in old person with osteopaenic bone [7, 8]. The main target of the surgeon is fracture reduction, preventing soft and bone tissues damages as much as possible. It is difficult to anatomically restore the cartilage surface using a mini invasive technique. Different methods and cancellous bone elevation instruments have been described, passing through a metaphysal cortex window [21]. Balloon tibioplasty, after a correct learning curve, may be a useful tool to facilitate the reduction of selected depressed tibial plateau fractures.

CONFLICT OF INTEREST

The author confirms that author has no conflict of interest to declare for this publication.

ACKNOWLEDGEMENTS

Declared none.

REFERENCES

[1]   Schatzker J, Tile M. The Rationale of Operative Fracture Care. 3rd. Berlin, Germany: Springer Verlag 2005; pp. 3-590.

[2]   Marsh JL, Slongo TF, Agel J, *et al*. Fracture and dislocation classification compendium - 2007: Orthopaedic Trauma Association classification, database and outcomes committee. J Orthop Trauma 2007; 21(10) (Suppl.): S1-S133.
[http://dx.doi.org/10.1097/00005131-200711101-00001] [PMID: 18277234]

[3]   Ballmer FT, Hertel R, Nötzli HP. Treatment of tibial plateau fractures with small fragment internal fixation: a preliminary report. J Orthop Trauma 2000; 14(7): 467-74.

[http://dx.doi.org/10.1097/00005131-200009000-00002] [PMID: 11083608]

[4]   Rasmussen PS. Tibial condylar fractures. Impairment of knee joint stability as an indication for surgical treatment. J Bone Joint Surg Am 1973; 55(7): 1331-50.
[PMID: 4586086]

[5]   Koval KJ, Helfet DL. Tibial plateau fracture, evaluation and treatment. J Am Acad Orthop Surg 1995; 3(2): 86-94.
[PMID: 10790657]

[6]   Roberts J. Fractures of the condyle of the tibia. J Bone Joint Surg Am 1968; 50: 1505.
[PMID: 5722847]

[7]   Hsu CJ, Chang WN, Wong CY. Surgical treatment of tibial plateau fracture in elderly patients 2001.
[http://dx.doi.org/10.1007/s004020000145]

[8]   Gerich T, Blauth M, Witte F, Krettek C. Osteosynthesis of fractures of the head of the tibia in advanced age. A matched-pair analysis. Unfallchirurg 2001; 104(1): 50-6.
[http://dx.doi.org/10.1007/s001130050687] [PMID: 11381762]

[9]   Biyani A, Reddy NS, Chaudhury J, Simison AJ, Klenerman L. The results of surgical management of displaced tibial plateau fractures in the elderly. Injury 1995; 26(5): 291-7.
[http://dx.doi.org/10.1016/0020-1383(95)00027-7] [PMID: 7649642]

[10] Martin J, Marsh JL, Nepola JV, Dirschl DR, Hurwitz S, DeCoster TA. Radiographic fracture assessments: which ones can we reliably make? J Orthop Trauma 2000; 14(6): 379-85.
[http://dx.doi.org/10.1097/00005131-200008000-00001] [PMID: 11001410]

[11] Lawler LP, Corl FM, Fishman EK. Multi- and single detector CT with 3D volume rendering in tibial plateau fracture imaging and management. Crit Rev Computed Tomogr 2002; 43(4): 251-82.
[PMID: 12390012]

[12] Kode L, Lieberman JM, Motta AO, Wilber JH, Vasen A, Yagan R. Evaluation of tibial plateau fractures: efficacy of MR imaging compared with CT. AJR Am J Roentgenol 1994; 163(1): 141-7.
[http://dx.doi.org/10.2214/ajr.163.1.8010201] [PMID: 8010201]

[13] Schatzker J, McBroom R, Bruce D. The tibial plateau fracture. The Toronto experience 1968--1975. Clin Orthop Relat Res 1979; (138): 94-104.
[PMID: 445923]

[14] Hohl M. Tibial condylar fractures. J Bone Joint Surg Am 1967; 49(7): 1455-67.
[PMID: 6053707]

[15] Muller M. The comprehensive classification of long bones. In: Muller ME, Allgower M, Schneider R, Willenegger H, Eds. Manual of internal fixation. Berlin: Springer-Verlag 1995; pp. 118-58.

[16] Antonius Pizanis MD, Patric Garcia MD, Tim Pohlemann MD. 2012.

[17] Broome B, Mauffrey C, Statton J, Voor M, Seligson D. Inflation osteoplasty: *in vitro* evaluation of a new technique for reducing depressed intra-articular fractures of the tibial plateau and distal radius. J Orthop Traumatol 2012; 13(2): 89-95.
[http://dx.doi.org/10.1007/s10195-012-0185-z] [PMID: 22391944]

[18] Hahnhaussen J, Hak DJ, Weckbach S, Heiney JP, Stahel PF. Percutaneous inflation osteoplasty for

indirect reduction of depressed tibial plateau fractures. Orthopedics 2012; 35(9): 768-72.
[http://dx.doi.org/10.3928/01477447-20120822-04] [PMID: 22955384]

[19]　Ahrens P, Sandmann G, Bauer J, *et al.* Balloon osteoplasty--a new technique for reduction and stabilisation of impression fractures in the tibial plateau: a cadaver study and first clinical application. Int Orthop 2012; 36(9): 1937-40.
[http://dx.doi.org/10.1007/s00264-012-1592-8] [PMID: 22729698]

[20]　Jordan R, Hao J, Fader R, Gibula D, Mauffrey C. Study protocol: trial of inflation osteoplasty in the management of tibial plateau fractures. Eur J Orthop Surg Traumatol 2014; 24(5): 647-53.
[http://dx.doi.org/10.1007/s00590-013-1260-8] [PMID: 23801029]

[21]　Rossi R, Castoldi F, Blonna D, Marmotti A, Assom M. Arthroscopic treatment of lateral tibial plateau fractures: a simple technique. Arthroscopy 2006; 22(6): 678.e1-6.
[http://dx.doi.org/10.1016/j.arthro.2005.09.028] [PMID: 16762710]

CHAPTER 7

Open Reduction and Internal Fixation of Tibial Plateau Fractures

Robert Barbin, Sridhar Vijayan, Narlaka Jayasekera [*] and **Matthew J Alfredson**

Department of Orthopaedics and Traumatology, Gold Coast University Hospital, Southport, Queensland, Australia

Abstract: Surgical fixation of tibial plateau fractures is technically challenging, carrying significant risks of complications for both patient and surgeon. A detailed understanding of the knee joint, coupled with classification of tibial plateau fractures, allows for accurate pre-operative planning and appropriate patient selection, resulting in the best possible outcome for patients. Open reduction and internal fixation of such fractures is done with the aim of restoring alignment, native articular surface of the knee, preventing early onset osteoarthritis. This chapter will explore the various surgical approaches described when approaching the tibial plateau, outlining the merits and drawbacks of each when undertaking open reduction and internal fixation of tibial plateau fractures.

Keywords: Approach, Fixation, Open, Osteosynthesis, Plateau fracture, Reduction.

CLASSIFICATION OF FRACTURES

Accurate classification of tibial plateau fractures allows for consistent clinical communication among surgeons, and appropriate formulation of treatment plans. Classification systems allow for documentation of soft-tissue damage, fracture location and extension pattern, all helping to guide treatment and the most appropriate surgical approach [1].

[*] **Correspondence author Narlaka Jayasekera:** Registrar, Trauma & Orthopaedics, Gold Coast University Hospital, 1 Hospital Boulevard Southport, Queensland 4215, Australia; Tel: +61455826899; E-mail: narlaka@me.com

Francesco Atzori and Luigi Sabatini (Eds)

The most common classification system used is the Schatzker classification [2].

Schatzker Type I

Schatzker Type I fractures are involving the lateral tibial plateau, resulting in a wedge shaped fragment displacing laterally and downwards [2, 3].

Schatzker Type II

Schatzker Type II fractures involve a wedge split from the lateral tibial plateau, combined with a comminuted fracture of the plateau with metaphyseal bony depression [2, 3].

Schatzker Type III

Schatzker Type III fractures are central depression fractures of the tibial articular surface, with an intact lateral cortex [2, 3].

Schatzker Type IV

Schatzker type IV is a fracture of the medial tibial plateau, either a split wedge fragment or a depressed comminuted fracture. Type IV fractures can also involve the tibial spine, and are associated with neurovascular compromise and ligamentous damage of the knee [2, 3].

Schatzker Type V

Schatzker Type V fractures represent bicondylar fractures involving the medial and lateral tibial plateau, and may involve the intercondylar area [2, 3].

Schatzker Type VI

Schatzker VI fracture is a bicondylar tibial plateau fracture, however there is dissociation of the diaphysis from the metaphysis. This type of fracture is associated with significant articular surface disruption and soft tissue damage [2, 3].

PRE-OPERATIVE CONSIDERATIONS

There are few circumstances in which immediate surgery is indicated for a tibial plateau fracture. However, such cases include open fractures, vascular compromise and the presence of compartment syndrome [4]. In the absence of these, surgical planning is dictated by the extent of soft-tissue damage. Physical examination, and when indicated further detailed imaging with Computed Tomography, are core components of pre-operative planning [1].

INTRA-OPERATIVE CONSIDERATIONS

Surgeon preference dictates patient positioning on the operating table. Typically, the patient is supine, unless a posterior approach is indicated [2]. A high riding tourniquet is placed on the thigh. The knee is flexed to at least 30° or can be left "hanging" off the table, allowing for release of the collateral ligamentous structures [1, 3, 4].

The use of a C-arm image intensifier intra-operatively is common practice, allowing for assessment of fracture reduction and implant placement. The C-arm image is typically placed on the contra-lateral side and should be sterile prepped prior to commencing surgery [1]. Concurrent arthroscopy can be considered, as it enables direct visualization of the meniscus and articular surface of the tibia. A femoral distractor may be utilized for surgical reduction of tibial plateau fractures, allowing for up to 0.5-1.0cm distraction of the joint. Manual traction is also used, but requires additional assistants, and would not provide an accurate fracture reduction and stable surgical field [1, 4].

Implant choice is vast and varied in the current market. Commonly, 'L' and 'T' plates are used in surgical fixation of both lateral and medial plateau fractures with cannulated screws [5]. Recent contoured plate designs facilitate cortical screw usage in locking and non-locking systems, allowing for support in comminuted fractures of the articular surface [4, 5]. Complex high energy fractures involving the metaphysis may require a bridging plate when fixing the lateral or medial plateau, to achieve adequate fixation of the condyles to the shaft of the tibia [6].

SURGICAL APPROACHES
Anterolateral

The anterolateral approach is commonly used to perform open reduction and internal fixation of a Schatzker Type I tibial plateau fracture. It allows direct exposure of the lateral aspect of the lateral tibial plateau, which is commonly involved in high and low energy injuries [1, 7]. Typically a standard straight incision will be used, beginning approximately 1-2 cm proximal to the joint line in the mid-axillary line. This incision is angled toward the lateral border of the anterior tibial crest and travels across Gerdy's Tubercle, dissecting the iliotibial bands in line with its fibers [4, 7].

Once an incision has been made, the musculature of the anterior compartment is dissected off its fascia and is mobilized from the metaphysis toward Gerdy's Tubercle [1, 4]. Dissection of the lateral extra-articular tissue should continue posteriorly to the proximal tibiofibular joint [1, 7]. This allows the surgeon to assess the integrity of the meniscus and isolate the meniscus from the fracture exposing the articular surface. The meniscus is reattached at the end of the surgery. When indicated, a femoral distractor should then be applied in the distal lateral femur and tibial shaft in a way that it will not disrupt the images of the C-arm [1].

The fracture of the lateral plateau should now be mobile and accessible. At this point the fragment should be cleaned of any early callus and organizing haematoma to identify the fracture fragments clearly allowing for adequate reduction. The surgeon may insert K-wires to isolate the fragment temporarily allowing for further surgical intervention to proceed [1, 7].

Posteromedial

The posteromedial approach is best utilized for medial tibial plateau fractures or bicondylar fractures of a high-energy injury. With the hip abducted and externally rotated and the knee flexed to 90°, a straight incision is made from the medial epicondyle to the posteromedial edge of the tibia [7]. This incision should carefully avoid the saphenous vein and saphenous nerve. The pes anserinus is then identifiable and should be moved anteriorly while the gastrocnemius should be moved posteriorly. The popliteus muscle should be cut and detached. This allows visualization of the fracture and appropriate debridement of any callus and haematoma, defining the fragmented bone [4].

Combinatory Anterolateral and Posteromedial Approach

For high-energy bicondylar tibial plateau fractures, seen in Schatzker V and VI, a combined approach is often utilized to allow access to both fractures, giving the surgeon an option for a double-plating ORIF (open reduction internal fixation) [8, 9]. This is an alternative to the anterior approach, which historically has shown significant wound breakdown and high complication rates [8]. This approach is suited for bicondylar fractures without severe soft-tissue disruption. Typically a posteromedial incision is applied for fixation of any medial fragments. This incision is closed once the fragment has been fixed and an anterolateral approach is utilized to then address the lateral fragment and fix the condyles to the shaft of the tibia [8].

Posterolateral Approach with Fibular Osteotomy

A posterolateral approach allows for access to posterolateral tibial plateau fractures that are difficult to access normally due to obstruction by strong ligamentous and tendinous structures of the popliteal corner [10]. With the patient in a lateral decubitus position, a 6 cm incision is made anterior to the biceps tendon to the fibular head, extending distally for a further 5cm [4, 10]. Then the common peroneal nerve is identified and protected. The deep fascia is exposed and the fascia lata is incised over the biceps femoris tendon. The common peroneal nerve is identified and exposed to the fibular head. Above the fibular head is the branch of the common peroneal nerve to the tibiofibular joint. This branch is transected [4, 10].

The common peroneal nerve is then exposed from the intermuscular septa of the peroneus muscles. Following this, the peroneus longus muscle is detached from the posterior septum, followed by exposure of the common peroneal nerve as it crosses into lateral compartment [4, 10]. The nerve is then released by dissection of the posterior septum. This procedure is repeated on the anterior septum to release the deep peroneal nerve, releasing the nerve from the surgical field [4, 10].

The fibular head is then dissected. The peroneus longus muscle is detached from the proximal fibula, thus exposing the fibular head. The surgeon then drills just lateral to the biceps tendon along the direction of the shaft. A curved osteotome is used to dissect the fibular neck approximately 2mm above the fibular nerve [4, 10]. The proximal tibiofibular joint capsule is released and the fibular head is then reflected proximally. Following incision of the synovial membrane, the coronary ligament of the knee is detached from the joint surface, allowing intra-articular view of the posterolateral tibia [4, 10].

Posterior

The posterior approach is utilized in a fracture that is purely isolated to the posterior portion of the tibial plateau involving both medial and lateral condyles [1].

A 'lazy S' incision is made starting proximo-medially, traversing over the popliteal crease, and extending over the posterolateral tibial crest distally [4]. Longitudinal dissection of the popliteal fascia is performed, beginning over the gastrocnemius. The sural nerve and lesser saphenous vein are identified and followed proximally into the popliteal fossa, which directs the surgeon to the popliteal vein and tibial nerve [4]. Care should be taken not to damage the peroneal nerve. Further dissection is performed with care to separate vessels and nerves. Separating vessels and nerves allows access between them. The posterior capsule and arcuate ligament is exposed. Fracture fragments can then be visualized and managed with appropriate plate and screw fixation [4].

REDUCTION BY FRACTURE TYPE

Schatzker Type I

The typical approach for an isolated lateral plateau fracture would be an anterolateral approach. If the fracture is primarily posterior in the plateau, a posterolateral approach should be considered [5].

Once the incision has been made and soft-tissue has been mobilized, a lateral distraction force is applied, at times using a femoral distractor. The fracture should then be reduced and held with forceps percutaneously [1, 5]. It is important to realize that if proper reduction of the fragment is not achievable, it may be that the lateral meniscus is incarcerated in the fracture line. For this same reason it is recommended to obtain MRI (magnetic resonance imaging) after surgery if adequate reduction is not achieved [1, 4, 8]. If the surgeon is suspicious of a meniscal tear, arthroscopic evaluation of the meniscus can be performed and subsequent open reduction and internal fixation of the fracture can be considered in cases of detached or trapped meniscus [4].

Adequate reduction of a Schatzker I is usually obtained with use of two to three lag screws. In fractures that are particularly comminuted where it is difficult to adequately reduce the fracture, or if there is significant osteoporosis, additional use of a lateral buttress plate with two to three lag screws should be considered. The leads author's general preference is to plate Schatzker I fractures. This provides an "antiglide" function and prevents displacement of the fragment distally [1, 8].

Schatzker Type II

In Schatzker II injuries, there can be varying degrees of articular surface depression. Proper pre-operative planning will require imaging studies to appreciate the degree of articular surface depression for any Schatzker Type II Case. Poor outcomes of Schatzker Type II Injuries are generally due to failure correct articular surface depression [9, 11].

For a Schatzker Type II, the location of a depressed articular surface is usually central or anterior, making the fracture ideally exposed with an anterolateral approach [11]. Once a submeniscal arthrotomy has been completed, the lateral meniscotibial ligament is incised transversely and stay-sutures are used to elevate the meniscus. Once the meniscus is lifted and the articular surface is visible, it is ideal to apply a varus force to the flexed knee to allow adequate visualization of the joint surface [4].

The impacted fragment is then reduced using one of two different techniques. The first technique is to wedge the fracture fragment open if the condylar fracture line is visualized. When the impacted fragments are visualized, the fracture can be disimpacted and elevated by a disimpactor inserted from below. When appropriate disimpaction is achieved, and the articular surface is restored, the fracture is temporarily stabilized by Kirschner wires [1]. It is important to note that disimpaction from below is preferable to elevating the fragment through the joint, so as to avoid production of loose osteochondral fragments [4].

By elevating the depressed fragment of bone, a defect is created in the metaphysis that needs to be grafted [1, 4]. Once the graft has been placed, the lateral condyle split is reduced and held together with forceps. The lateral wedge can then be fixed with a periarticular buttress plate with lag screws. Three to four 3.5mm screws can be placed horizontally to support the osteochondral fragments [5]. The meniscotibial ligament is then repaired.

The second common approach for fixation of split-depressed fractures is to reduce the lateral condyle first and hold it with forceps and reduce the depressed osteochondral fragment by using a cortical window [1]. This is useful in cases where the condylar fracture line is not immediately visible as an alternative to further dissection of the anterior compartment musculature. The window is created by drilling multiple small holes into the cortex and connecting them with use of an osteotome [1]. An impactor is used to impact into the cortex, and under fluoroscopic guidance, engages the depressed fracture from below. Graft material must be placed continuously beneath the fracture to elevate the fragment. Once the joint surface is restored a peri-articular plate is applied and raft screws are placed [1, 4].

Schatzker Type III

Schatzker III fractures are more commonly due to low-energy injuries in elderly patients. Surgical management is only indicated in cases where joint instability is evident. In many cases arthroscopic reduction is the primary treatment option, however in some cases an additional buttress plate may be required to achieve stability of osteochondral fragments. In any case, arthroscopy to assist adequate reduction is recommended [4, 11].

A metaphyseal cortical window is produced and a bone void filler is inserted allowing the surgeon to bone graft and subsequently elevate the depressed fragment. The cortical window can be on the medial tibial metaphysis for depressed fractures that are anteriorly situated, and on the lateral tibial metaphysis for posterolateral fractures. In some cases, particularly in insufficiency fractures, the use of a lateral plateau plate and a raft of screws can be utilized to support the fragments once elevated [1].

Schatzker Type IV

Schatzker type IV – VI result from high-energy trauma. They are usually comminuted fractures and are typically associated with significant soft-tissue injury including LCL tearing or an avulsion of the fibular head, and avulsion of the ACL. The rate of neurovascular compromise is significantly higher in Schatzker IV – VI fractures, as well as compartment syndrome, which occurs within hours of sustaining the initial injury [8, 9]. Due to the significant soft-tissue injury, complete recovery by means other than surgery does not guarantee great outcome [6]. The extent of soft-tissue injury also dictates the required approach for fixation of these fracture types. If the fracture is more medially situated a posteromedial approach may be required. If the fracture is more posteriorly situated, a posterior approach may be more ideal. The prone positioning may be of significant advantage when addressing an isolated posteromedial fracture as fracture reduction is facilitated by extension of the knee. This decision is guided by pre-operative imaging and physical examination [4, 11, 1].

Depending on the approach, the incision is required to reach as close to the apex of the condylar fracture line as possible. Once the fracture has been visualized, fixation is achieved with a buttress plate [5]. The plate is ideally situated in contact with the entire metaphyseal surface. To achieve this, the entire pes anserinus may need to be elevated with the superficial portion of medial collateral ligament [5]. Care should be taken not to trap soft-tissue beneath the plate. Any small avulsion fragments of the intercondylar area should be fixed with a small screw or sutures placed through drill holes [4].

Schatzker Type V – VI

Schatzker's V and VI are the highest energy fractures and are associated with the greatest amount of soft-tissue injury and neurovascular complications. It is suggested that open bicondylar tibial plateau fractures be managed with external fixation [12]. The reason for this is the significant soft-tissue damage and high energy injuries are more susceptible to complications and wound infection. Closed injuries are suitable for open reduction and internal fixation. The initial treatment should be to apply a bridging external fixator to allow time for the soft-tissues to settle and the proper assessment and planning for definitive fracture management. Distraction will also improve the alignment of the condyles [12].

A dual incision and plating technique is used, where fixation of the medial column is the primary step [5]. A Posteromedial approach is used initially [12]. The dissection of subperiosteal tissue is limited by the fracture edge. Once the fracture component has been identified, the fragment is held with forceps. Any articular depression at this point should be addressed by utilizing techniques similar to those outlined for split depression fractures; either through disimpaction from below the fracture or through a submetaphyseal cortical window [4]. A plate is applied to achieve fixation of the medial plateau. Some surgeons prefer a small fragment reduction plate while others prefer locked reconstruction plates [5, 12].

The lateral plateau is then attended *via* anterolateral approach. At this point a femoral distractor should be applied and there should be reduction of the lateral condyle and the metaphyseal/diaphyseal fracture [4, 12]. Any subchondral defects are then bone grafted, again in a fashion similar to those outlined in the Schatzker II/III repairs. As with split-depressed fracture, a plate is used for stabilization and screws are used to support articular comminution. In many high-energy tibial plateau fractures, the lateral plateau is more comminuted than the medial plateau [12]. For this reason, a buttress plate is utilized on the lateral plateau [5]. Once the condyles have been reduced, extension of the incision in an extraperiosteal fashion allows exposure of lateral submetaphyseal and shaft regions. A buttress plate allows fixation of the shaft to the condyle. It should be noted that in most of these types of fractures, dual plating is only ideal for those without significant soft-tissue injury [12]. In cases with significant soft-tissue injury, external fixation is the ideal treatment option or a combined internal and external fixation technique [12].

COMPLICATIONS

Tibial plateau fixations have previously been known to carry considerable complication rates, particularly in the setting of high-energy, such as Schatzker IV – VI fractures. This has improved with advancements in surgical approach and pre-operative assessment and planning. The risk of infection may be reduced by delaying surgery to allow soft-tissues to heal and swelling to settle. Alternative incisions can be used to avoid areas with significant soft-tissue damage [4, 11].

Infectious complications are still reported in high-energy fractures. Barei *et al.* reported complications of high-energy fractures fixed with internal dual incision and plating technique. Of 83 patients, 7 developed deep-wound infections, and a statistical association was drawn between vascular injuries requiring vascular reconstruction and deep wound infection. This is reflected in other studies that show similar infection rates regardless of the fixation method [8].

Non-union can occur following these procedures. Barei *et al.* found one patient requiring further management for non-union in his study of 83 patients [8]. Manidakis *et al.* studied 125 patients who sustained tibial plateau fractures and underwent fixation. Their studied showed a non-union rate of 1.6%. Treatment options for non-union include bone grafting, revision of fixation and total knee arthroplasty [9].

Osteoarthritis is another common complication of tibial plateau fractures and non-operative treatment. In Manidakis' study of 125 patients, 33 developed osteoarthritis with varying levels of pain. Furthermore, five patients required TKR due to significant collapse and OA [9].

Contractures can result from surgical intervention. This is of particular concern if a posterior approach is utilized. Proper post-operative involvement of physiotherapy and mobilization planning is paramount in preventing development of contractures [4].

SUMMARY

Tibial plateau fractures remain an evolving area of orthopaedic surgery. The most important part in the management of tibial plateau surgery is the assessment and pre-planning stage. Proper care for planning will direct the surgeon to utilise the most suited surgical approach, technique and implant, and to do so at the most appropriate time. While open reduction remains the mainstay of treatment for tibial plateau fractures, new surgical techniques continue to introduce opportunities for intervention with different outcomes. For now, open reduction and internal fixation is shown to be an effective option in the management of tibial plateau fractures in terms of restoration of knee joint alignment and anatomy and prevention of progression to post-traumatic osteoarthritis.

CONFLICT OF INTEREST

The author confirms that author has no conflict of interest to declare for this publication.

ACKNOWLEDGEMENTS

Declared none.

REFERENCES

[1]   Watson JT, Wiss DA. Tibial plateau fractures: Open reduction internal fixation. D Wiss, Master Techniques in Orthopaedic Surgery: Fractures . Lippincott: Williams & Wilkins 2006; pp. 408-37.

[2]   Schatzker J, McBroom R, Bruce D. The tibial plateau fracture. The Toronto experience 1968--1975. Clin Orthop Relat Res 1979; (138): 94-104.
        [PMID: 445923]

[3]   Langford JR, Jacofsky DJ, Haidukewych GJ. Tibial plateau fractures. In: Scott N, Ed. Insall & Scott Surgery of the Knee . Churchill Livingstone 2011; pp. 773-85.

[4]   Cole PA, Lafferty PM, Levy BA, Watson JT. Tibial plateau fractures. In: Browner B D, Ed. Skeletal Trauma: Basic Science, Management, and Reconstruction. University of California: Saunders 2014; pp. 1937-2015.

[5]   Ebraheim NA, Sabry FF, Haman SP. Open reduction and internal fixation. Orthopaedics 2004; 27(12): 1281-7.
        [PMID: 15633959]

[6]   Ziran BH, Hooks B, Pesantez R. Complex fractures of the tibial plateau. J Knee Surg 2007; 20(1): 67-77.
        [PMID: 17288092]

[7]   Manidakis N, Dosani A, Dimitriou R, Stengel D, Matthews S, Giannoudis P. Tibial plateau fractures: functional outcome and incidence of osteoarthritis in 125 cases. Int Orthop 2010; 34(4): 565-70.
        [http://dx.doi.org/10.1007/s00264-009-0790-5] [PMID: 19440710]

[8]   Barei DP, Nork SE, Mills WJ, Henley MB, Benirschke SK. Complications associated with internal fixation of high-energy bicondylar tibial plateau fractures utilizing a two-incision technique. J Orthop Trauma 2004; 18(10): 649-57.
[http://dx.doi.org/10.1097/00005131-200411000-00001] [PMID: 15507817]

[9]   Raykov D, Ivanov S, Apostolov P. Tibial plateau fractures - Standard and specific surgical approaches. Scripta Scientifica Medica 2013; pp. 74-81.

[10]   Yu B, Han K, Zhan C, Zhang C, Ma H, Su J. Fibular head osteotomy: a new approach for the treatment of lateral or posterolateral tibial plateau fractures. Knee 2010; 17(5): 313-8.
[http://dx.doi.org/10.1016/j.knee.2010.01.002] [PMID: 20163966]

[11]   Fenton P, Porter K. Tibial plateau fractures: A review. Trauma 2011; 13(3): 181-7.
[http://dx.doi.org/10.1177/1460408610396422]

[12]   Prasad GT, Kumar TS, Kumar RK, Murthy GK, Sundaram N. Functional outcome of Schatzker type V and VI tibial plateau fractures treated with dual plates. Indian J Orthop 2013; 47(2): 188-94.
[http://dx.doi.org/10.4103/0019-5413.108915] [PMID: 23682182]

CHAPTER 8

Damage Control Orthopaedics and the Role of External Fixation in Tibial Plateau Fractures

Daniele Santoro*

University of Turin, Unit of Traumatology, C.T.O. Hospital, Turin, Italy

Abstract: The plateau tibial fracture is a challenging pathology where associated lesions can complicate by far the fracture treatment. External fixation could be a valuable option, both in the emergency stabilization and in the definitive synthesis, especially when general or local patient's conditions demand for a tissue sparing approach. This chapter is divided in two, the first part talks about the indications and the technical rules of the bridging external fixators and the clinical applications of Damage Control Orthopedics (DCO) to tibial plateau fractures. The second part is focused on those complex (because of the soft tissue envelope conditions or the fracture pattern) lesions that could take advantage of a definitive treatment based on the external fixation, more frequently circular. Technical and mechanical characteristics, indications, surgical application, pros and cons of the circular frames are described.

Keywords: Damage control, External fixation, Fractures, Reduction, Soft tissue injuries, Tibial plateau.

INTRODUCTION

The knee joint and the tibial plateau, differently from the hip, but similarly to the ankle, lie under a relatively poor soft tissues coverage [1].

Fractures of the plateau can be up to major trauma, such as motorbike accidents or falls from height, as to lower energy traumas, such as the knee twisting very common in skiers.

* **Correspondence author Daniele Santoro:** University of Turin, Unit of Traumatology, C.T.O. Hospital, *Via* Gianfranco Zuretti 29, 10126 Turin, Italy; Tel: +3901169331; E-mail: daniele.santoro01@gmail.com

Francesco Atzori and Luigi Sabatini (Eds)

The conditions of the soft tissue surroundings are very important in planning the therapy strategies. Very often the fracture is open, but even when it is closed, the poor conditions of the soft tissue envelope can be a severe threat to the functional outcome. The incidence of open tibial plateau fracture appears to be relatively low if considering all fracture patterns (4.8% in a revision of 8,426 patients with monolateral tibial plateau), but it can increase dramatically when we focus on more challenging casuistries, depending on high energy traumas (13 open fractures out of 31, grade-IIIA according to the Gustilo-Anderson classification, being the remaining 18 closed fractures characterized by severe soft tissue lesions, Tscherne and Oestern grade 2/3, in a recent series) (Figs. **1, 2**) [2, 3].

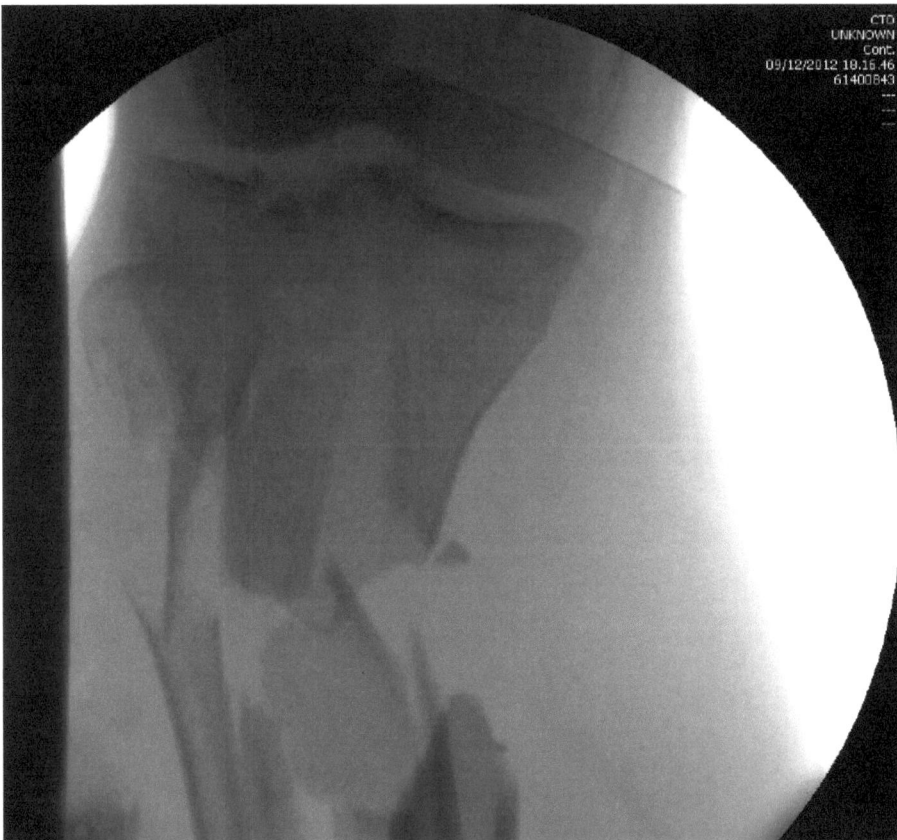

Fig. (1). N. C., male, 30 yrs., right leg badly crushed by a car in motorcycle accident (December the 9th 2012): severe bone loss (about 9 cm), skin degloving, huge soft tissue mangling (open fracture Oestern and Tscherne grade III or Gustilo-Anderson IIIA), tibial plateau fracture AO 41.B3.1 or Schatzker II (split with depression). AP view.

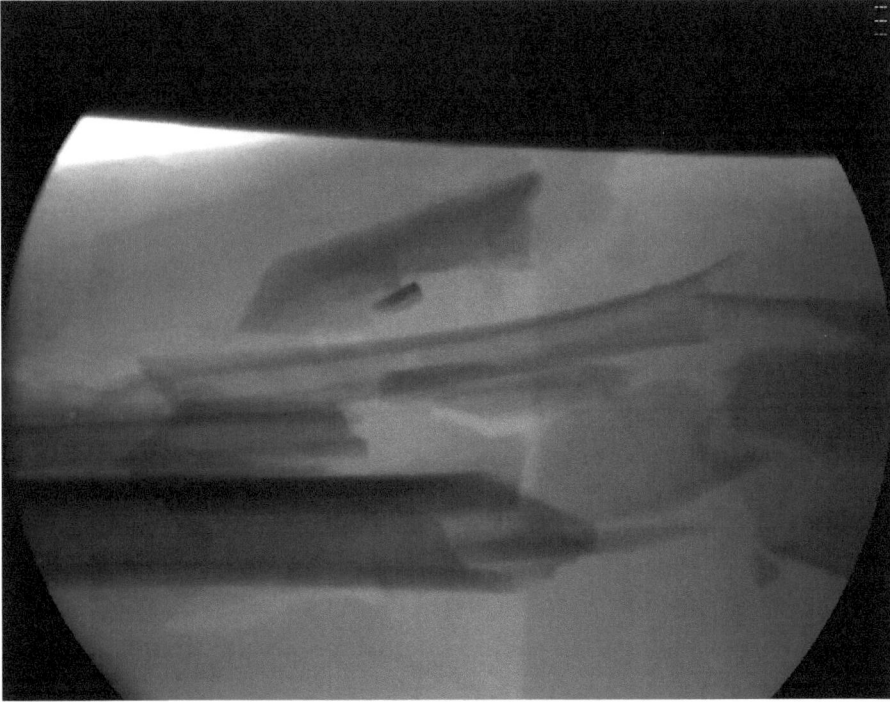

Fig. (2). Lat. view.

When the trauma energy is higher, there is the possibility for the tibial plateu fractures to be associated with other injuries (53/239, 22.6% in a Brazilian casuistry) [4].

Tibial plateau fractures, closed or open, especially when involving the medial side (Schatzker IV/VI), represent a risk factor for arterial injuries [5]. Serious implications of these fractures could be the nerve injuries, especially the peroneal nerve, and the compartment syndrome [6, 7].

The aim of the surgical treatment is the functional recovery of the painless knee function through the anatomical reconstruction of the joint surface and the axial and torsional restoration of the tibial shaft. The amount of residual acceptable articular depression and dyaphiseal dislocation is still far to be widespread accepted [8].

Open reduction and internal fixation (ORIF), ensuring precocious motion through a stable synthesis, are considered to be the gold standard of the surgical treatment. Sadly this therapeutic approach is burdened with a heavy load of possible early or delayed complications: superficial/deep infections, knee stiffness, post-traumatic arthritis, nonunions, chronic pain. Old casuistries showed frightening infection rates, up to 80% in patients who underwent ORIF, while more recent and more extended reviews have shown less dire data (4.2%) [9, 10]. Open fractures have demonstrated to be more prone to post-surgical infections when treated by means of ORIF, where the incidence of infection is 5.3% for a closed fracture, 14.3% for Gustilo-Anderson (G-A) grade 1, 40% for G-A grade 2, 50% for G-A grade 3 [10, 11]. Prolonged surgical time performing ORIF can increase the risk for a deep post-surgical infection [11, 12].

Beyond the injury "personality", the patient's anamnesis could lead the surgeon to different therapeutic options. Diabetes mellitus has shown to be a condition that increases the risk for superficial or deep infections, considering orthopaedic surgery in general, even if, when talking of ORIF of the tibial plateau fractures, its influence on the infection rate and the short-term functional results is controversial [13 - 15]. A high ASA (America Society of Anaesthesiologists) score classification seems to predispose to adverse events [9].

Age should be an important issue in planning strategies, because a very aggressive surgery could be a dangerous option when the functional needs are low.

It is evident that the soft tissues envelope, together with the possible associated lesions, the patient's age and his/her past pathological conditions are not a minor subject, but they are features the surgeon should carefully focus on.

Talking about the external fixation in the treatment of articular fractures, the subject should be divided in at least two main chapters, being the first the urgency external frame bridging the femur to the tibia as a stabilization tool (not very differently from a splint cast), according to the Damage Control Orthopaedics (DCO) rules, and the second an approach to the tibial plateau fractures with the external fixator, more often circular, as the definitive treatment.

The temporary external fixator can either be the first step of a traditional ORIF strategy, that will be performed when the acute inflammation has regressed, or the beginning of an "all ex-fix" protocol: the temporary fixator will be changed with a circular one as soon as soft tissue conditions and the availability of an Ilizarov-trained surgeon will allow for.

THE ROLE OF TEMPORARY EXTERNAL FIXATOR IN URGENT STABILIZATION

The role of the urgency bridging external fixator in the DCO has been deeply investigated and, nowadays, the non-invasive quick stabilization of fractures, both diaphiseal and articular, in unstable patients is a standard procedure in many trauma centres (Fig. **3**) [16 - 23].

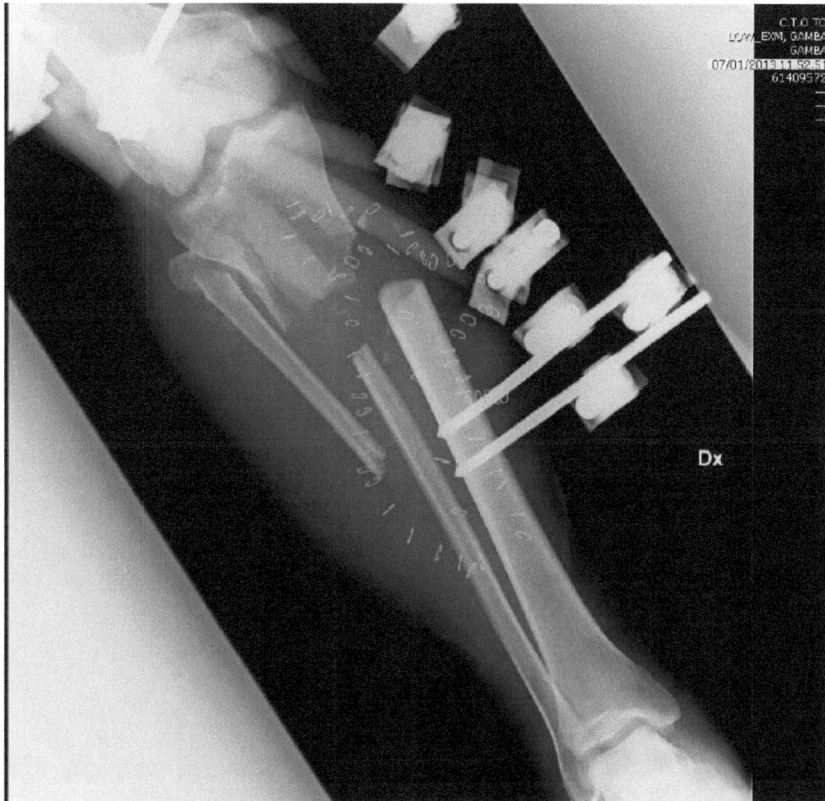

Fig. (3). Emergency: bridging exfix, thorough debridement, bone resection, shortening, after 10 days plastic surgery coverage was performed.

Some authors have tried to take those principles of minimal invasive philosophy from the early life saving procedures to a strategy oriented to get the best from a traumatized joint. An early bony stabilization by means of a spanning external fixator is worthy in preserving at its best the soft tissue coverage, to preserve the limb length, to protect the joint during the deinflammation phase. Deglovings, severe abrasions, muscle infarctions, crashing injuries can be as dangerous and ominous as a severe bone exposition actually is [24]. The temporary bridging optimises the analgesia, the nursing, the wound care (even in case of any second look), while being helpful in protecting a contingent vascular suture, stabilizing a limb when fasciotomies have been performed for compartment syndrome, eventually safeguarding for the early period an internal fixation after the definitive internal synthesis has been carried out [25].

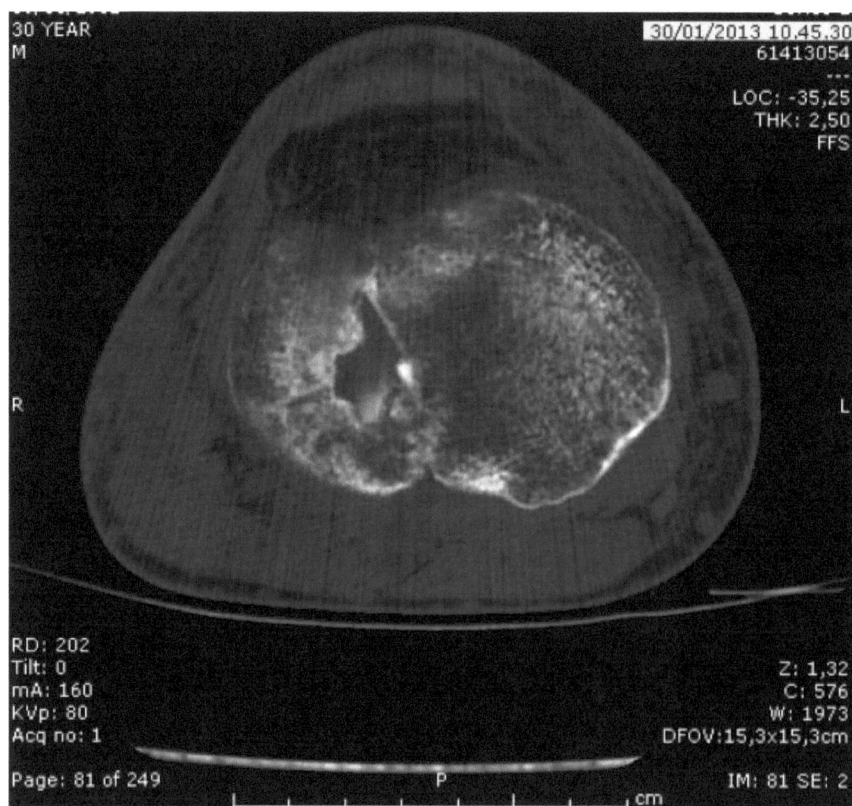

Fig. (4). CT-scan for definitive surgery planning. Axial view.

Some Authors, having observed a rate of complications surprisingly low when

ORIF was carried out after the bridging fixator was placed in emergency, have proposed a staged treatment protocol, where the ex-fix is the first step, allowing for soft tissue care and recovery, followed by the traditional internal fixation [26, 27].

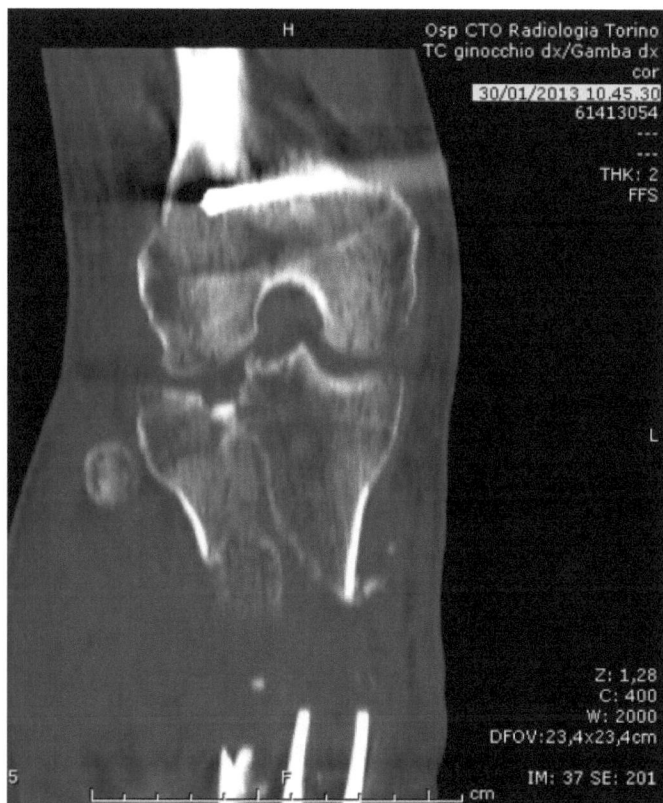

Fig. (5). CT-scan for definitive surgery planning. Coronal view.

The spanning fixator, as well as the "systemic" DCO, has proven itself to be a relatively safe, if properly conducted, procedure, without affecting the functional outcome [28, 29]. Furthermore, this approach, in association with the administration of a prophylaxis based on low molecular weight heparin administration, showed an incidence of deep venous thrombosis (DVT) comparable to that of historical series. It has been hypothesized that the limb length restoration together with the possibility of a prompt mobilization could prevent the establishment of DVT [30].

Concerning diagnosis and precise injury definition, the author's opinion is that in emergency CT scan is seldom useful, as an average trauma orthopaedic surgeon should be well trained in recognizing a tibial plateau fracture that would benefit from a urgent stabilization by the two traditional x-ray views. Anyway, as CT scan is mandatory in planning the definitive synthesis [24], this can be performed with no hurry after the bridging fixator is in place, the fracture realigned, the main fragments less impacted: this way the amount of information we will get from images is far more superior [31]. MRI can be helpful, but not essential and it is very seldom required (Figs. **4-7**) [24].

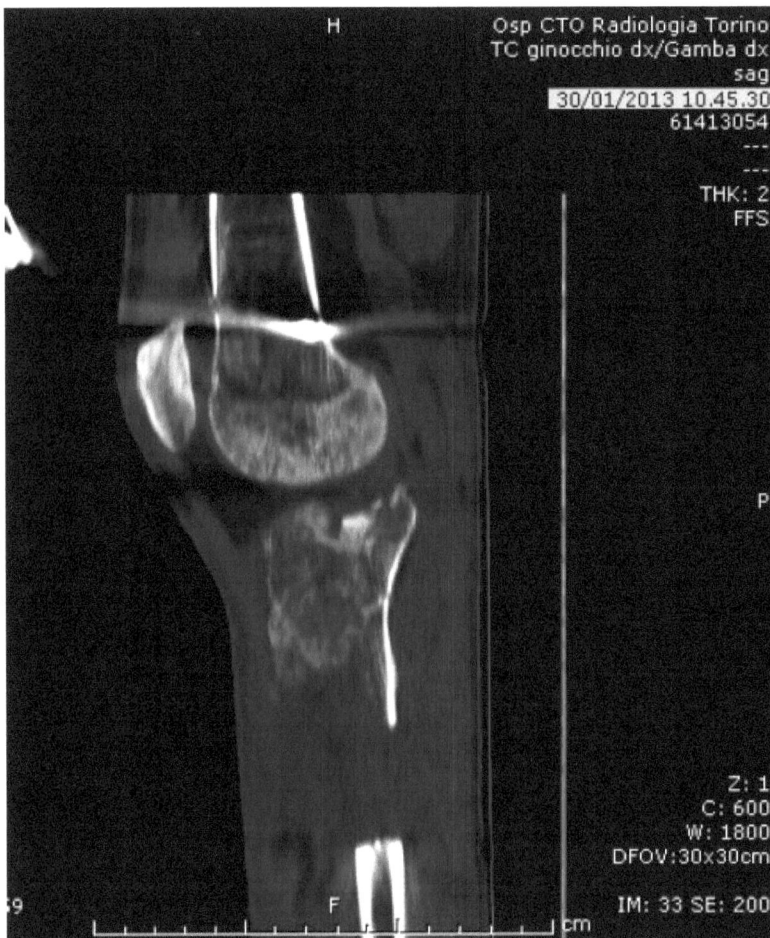

Fig. (6). CT-scan for definitive surgery planning. Sagittal view.

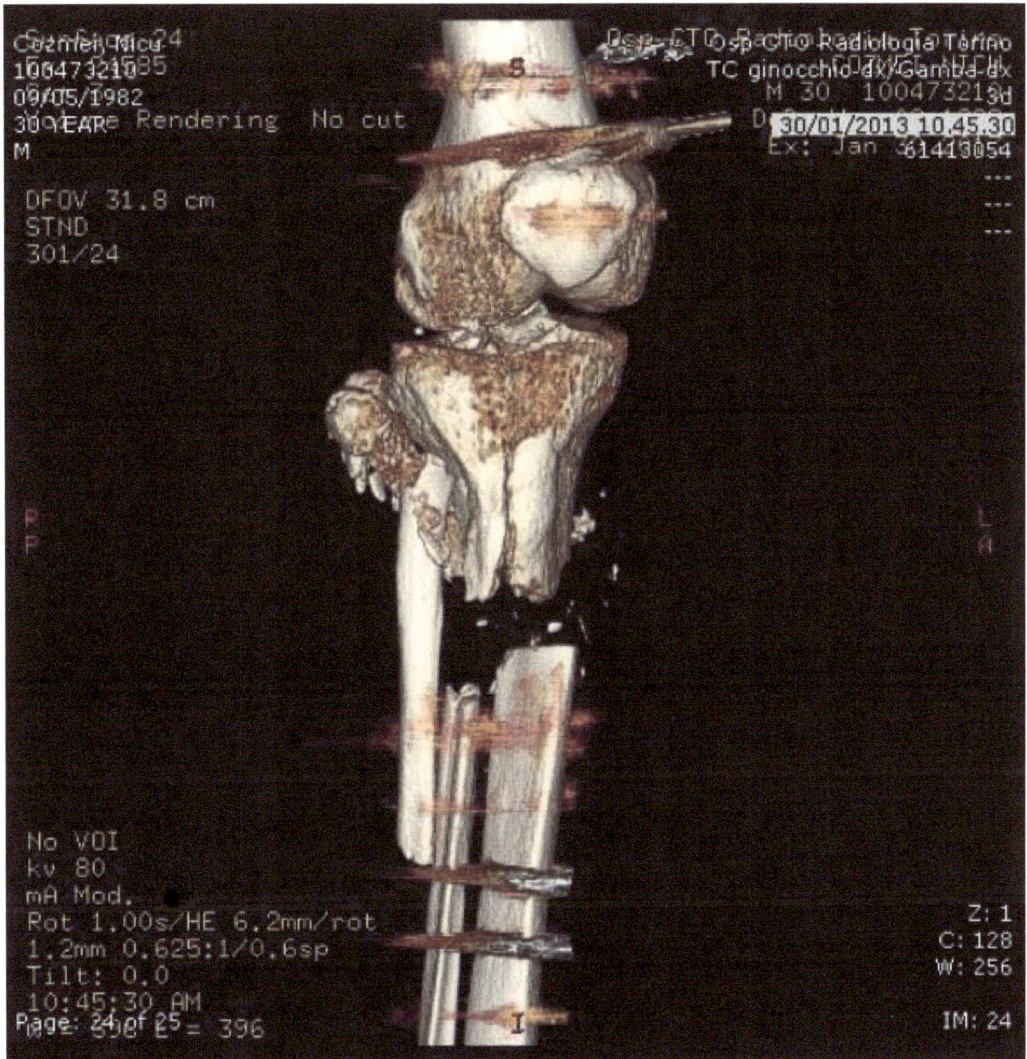

Fig. (7). CT-scan for definitive surgery planning. 3-D view.

Haidukewych, who introduced the concept of "portable traction", has conveniently written up a handy and readymade list of indications for urgent bridging fixator. As it is so synthetically and well expressed, I will simply cite it between quotation marks: <<tibial pilon fractures, tibial plateau fractures, distal femur fractures, open ankle [*and knee, a. e.*] dislocations, compartment syndromes with complex fractures, fracture blisters, severe abrasions, vascular injuries, multiple complex injuries in unstable, polytrauma patients, inability to

cast or splint due to vacuum assisted closures, augment internal fixation (small plates, osteoporotic bone), protect soft tissues after internal fixation, battlefield/mass casualty situations, intraoperative reduction tool>> [25]. I think every trauma orthopaedic surgeon should take this list in his/her pocket.

No commercial product has shown any significant advantage over another, so there is not any recommendation in this sense.

When bridging a tibial plateau fracture in emergency, few simple rules should be followed: the procedure should be fast, the screws must avoid to exceed too much the far cortex width (be aware of the possible anatomic structures in danger), their positions should not interfere with following planned surgical approaches, the construct must be stable, its building scheme should anticipate the needs for inspection, dressings, fasciotomies, possible second surgical looks.

The screws can be inserted anterior both in the femur and in the tibia, or antero-laterally in the femur and antero-medially in the tibia. Not more than two screws per segment is needed. The knee should be put in a slight flexed position (about 15°/20°). A mild traction is acted through the knee. All the commercial devices are modular and they are quite easy to be connected. When building a square-shaped frame, a good tip is to cross the square with an additional bar so the construct is stiffer [32].

Radiolucent bed and fluoroscopy C-arm can be helpful tools, but, in the Institution where I work, we have experienced the emergency bridging stabilization in the shock room of the trauma department without observing any particular complications: this can be an option when the patient is too unstable or when an operating room still busy or while waiting for pending diagnostic procedures (*i.e.* CT scan). It takes about 10-15 minutes, draping included, a little bit more advanced practical skill is needed, it can be performed without stopping resuscitation and other lifesaving procedures.

It has been observed that, in femur shaft fractures, when DCO is performed, the risk of contamination is higher if the ex-fix screws are kept in place for more than two weeks. Up to this, it would be desirable to convert the bridging fixator to an ORIF before this date [33]. As this is not always achievable, the importance of keeping the screws well far away from "safe zones", where the surgical approaches will be carried out, must be again underlined.

Nevertheless, the fear for an increase infection rate, because of the possible overlap between plates and former pin sites, appears to be not supported by evidence [34].

Perforating the diaphyseal bone, both with self-drilling screws or with bores, needs some caution. The over-perforation of the far cortex must be avoided because of the risk for coiling the anatomical structures on the other side. So, when the apex of the bore or of the screw touches the inner surface of the far cortex, we should stop drilling and lock a safety ring-shaped stop over the bore/screw at a distance of about the cortex width (5-10 mm) from the near end of the protection sleeve. Starting drilling again, the apex cannot perforate too further beyond the far cortex [35].

Bridging emergency external fixators have proven to be an easy and ready device also in those environments where resources are poor (small peripheral hospitals, developing countries, war areas). If the patient has to be referred to a more specialized setting, they are the right tool for the task, putting the patient in a better condition for the transfer, without compromising any further therapeutic option, allowing the referring hospital and the referential one to plan the logistics at its best [36 - 40].

THE ROLE OF CIRCULAR EXTERNAL FIXATOR IN THE DEFINITIVE TREATMENT OF THE TIBIAL PLATEAU FRACTURES

Plateau tibial fractures have come across as one of the battlefields of the orthopaedic scientific debate. Diagnosis is rightly considered to be the first step of a proper therapy. Sadly, it is a long way to share the same vision among surgeons concerning a comprehensive approach to the topic [31]. There are two main classifications for the fracture patterns, AO and Schatzker [24, 41, 42], plus sub-classifications [6], two classifications for open fractures, Gustilo-Anderson and Oestern-Tscherne [43, 44], the latter taking into account also the soft tissue injuries in closed fractures, some Authors focused on ligaments and on the joint instability [45], different follow-up scoring systems have been implemented, both patient- and clinician-based [46, 47, 48].

A significant inter-observer variability has been observed in evaluating x-rays and patients [31].

A recent study that reviewed literature and analyzed the 6-year follow-up of 82 patients by means of returned questionnaires, showed "fair" results in terms of general daily activities, but poorer if focused on sports. The same study outlined again the lack of knowledge when setting the cut-off for joint reduction, between what is acceptable and what is not. The energy of trauma is a major feature (the higher the energy, the poorer the outcome), together with age. However, age can be a misleading factor, where young patients often ask for more from their post-traumatic knee, while elderly population is easier to please [8].

Smoking reduces TGF-b1 in serum level, perhaps causing an impairment in the fracture healing [49]. Smoking has shown to be a predictor of deep surgical infection after tibial plateau fractures ORIF [9, 50].

The length of operative time [11] and the male sex, the increased ASA class, pulmonary disease [9], the diabetes mellitus [13 - 15] play their role in addressing functional results.

The number of controversies should not paralyse the surgeon, but the planning should be shifted from an abstract fracture, to a well defined case, where all the pathology features (fracture, exposure, soft tissue classifications, ligamentous asset, energy of the trauma), patient's age and genre, co-existing diseases (diabetes mellitus, neurological impairment, psychological status), habits (smoke), pre-trauma activities, functional needs, expectations are carefully evaluated and pondered.

The circular external fixation, very often associated to an open/miniopen internal reduction, of joint fractures is not a universal tool good for all the cases, but, when properly planned and carried out, it can be a handy and versatile technique, useful in fixing problems otherwise very complicated for the patient and demanding for the surgeon. The goal of a circular frame in such fractures is to optimise the soft tissue handling to the best articular reduction achievable.

In order to regain the perfect restoration, a tibial plateau fracture would be ideally assessed by huge multiple surgical approaches. Unfortunately the soft tissue envelope is very flimsy and can badly tolerate such aggressiveness [51]. The bone too has to be preserved from a too deep dissection that can cause necrosis [27, 52].

The unavailability of the medial side for an ORIF (exposition or comminution) prompted some Authors to reinforce the medial column with a monolateral frame, but this showed some problems in terms of stability and half pins infection [53]. The circular external frames, on the other side, have shown better mechanical features in terms of stability, bending, axial rigidity. They moreover offer the possibility of correcting some degrees of axial, rotational and translational malalignment, compression can be elicited through the metaphiseal fracture site [54].

A recent study, based on the comparison between a treatment with minimal invasive approach associated to a TSF circular frame and a traditional ORIF, found no correlations between the quality of the reduction and the 1-year follow-up functional result [55]. This seems to be partially in contradiction with the opposite statement of a group that re-evaluated a pure-ORIF casuistry where the better quality of articular reduction lead to a better function [56]. Probably, the answers are both true: when performing a minimal invasive surgery, the sparing of the soft tissues allows for an early mobilization, with a less affecting part played by the inflammation and the reaction to surgery.

In addressing a plateau tibial fracture, like in the majority of the joint injuries, the are two main issues: the joint surface restoration and the metaphiseal reduction.

A radiolucent bed is the starting point: it must be equipped with a stiff removable support that allows the knee to be flexed and pulled at the same time. Tackling the problem of joint fragmentation, the tibial plateau can be reduced by means of small approaches, through traditional more or less extensile incisions or indirectly with the help of some traction across the fracture site. To get the traction acting through the fracture, some grips over the femur are needed: in the easiest cases the manual force of the second operator pulling the flexed knee is sufficient, but sometimes this is not enough and a large distractor between one half pin in the femur and one in the tibia or a traditional trans-calcaneal traction (counterbalanced by the flexed knee) can be helpful. The collapse of the joint surface is rarely reduced by the sole traction and would be better addressed through the fracture line or through a small bone window opened by the surgeon at the anterior (lateral) cortex to allow a tamp or a Mayo scissor to push the fragments up [32, 57]. Some Authors suggest that small fragments may be manipulated with a K wire, as it was a joystick [58].

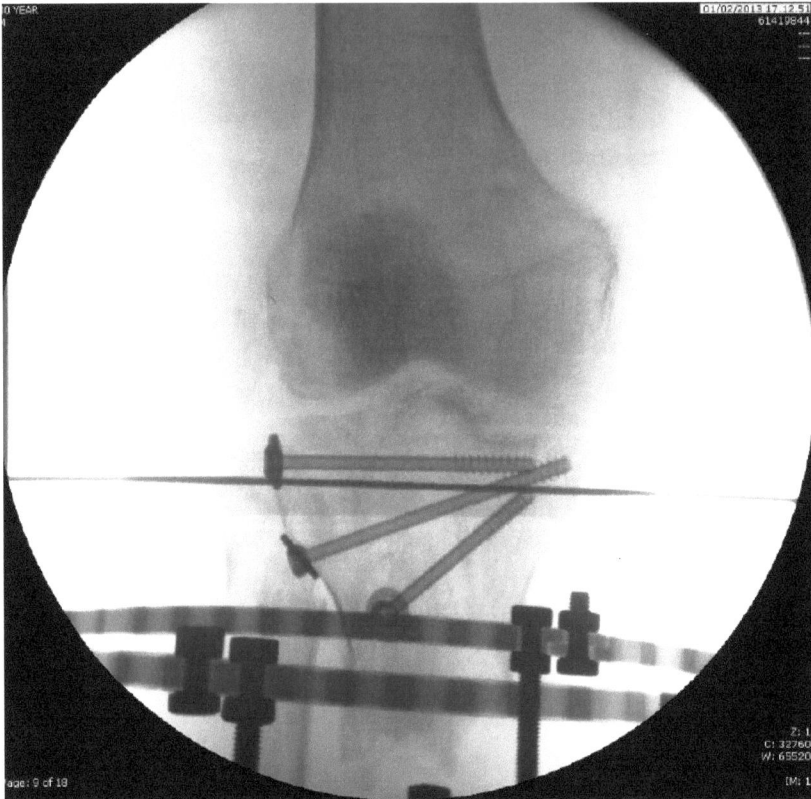

Fig. (8). Intra-operative images. Note the traditional screw-based ORIF for the tibial plateau, the first proximal wire, parallel to the joint line the treatment was performed 54 days after the trauma because of the soft tissue conditions. AP view.

If fracture lines run vertically (Schatzker I and V, less frequently IV and VI), the pelvis clamps or any big button-headed reduction clamp can be helpful tools [32]. The surgeon should avoid pointed skin necrosis by making small incisions where the clamp tips squeeze. Attention must be paid not to over-penetrate the bone with the clamps, especially in elderly patients.

When going through traditional/minimal invasive surgical arthrotomy, general rules of meniscus handling must be obeyed: this must be kindly detached from its distal insertion, tied to two suture wires, gently pulled up, ready for the reinsertion in the anatomical position at the end of the operation [59].

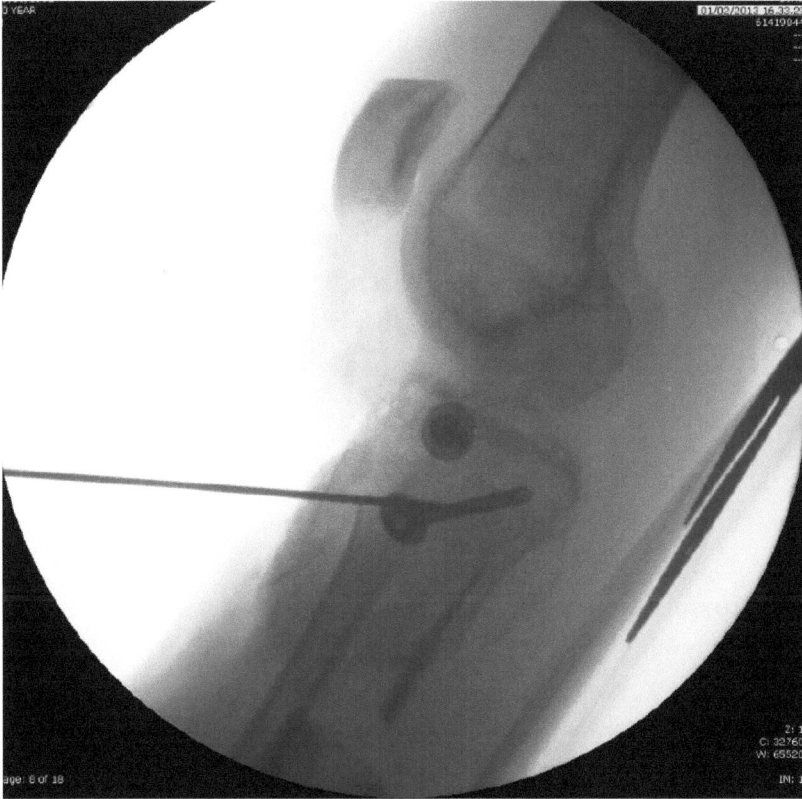

Fig. (9). Intra-operative images. Lat. view.

Cannulated screws (diameter from 4.0 mm up to 6.5 mm), inserted in the subcondral bone perpendicularly to the fracture lines as detected on the CT scan, could "lock" the fracture plateau. They can also bear a re-elevated fragment. When screws are not indicated, the reduction of the tibial plateau can be maintained by means of 2 olive wires acting reciprocally counterforce, both connected to the proximal ring [32, 57, 58, 60]. One of the two olive wires can transfix the proximal fibula, making the fibula head work as a buttress (Fig. **8, 9**) [60].

Once the articular reduction, by direct view or by fluoroscopy or by arthoscopic check [61], is satisfactory, the proximal/epiphyseal block needs to be assembled. The restored articular surface is the cornerstone for the insertion of the first wire: this one should be parallel/3° varus to the joint line [58]. In order to avoid the most proximal wire to transfix the capsule, the entrance point should be at least 14 mm distal to the joint line, thus reducing the septic arthritis risk (Fig. **8**) [62].

The most proximal ring is set by means of at least two crossing wires. The epiphyseal block gets its stability assembling a "tripod", a structure that prevents the reciprocal torsion between the ring and the bone. It can be assembled connecting with threaded rods the proximal ring to a more distal one, this latter united to the bone by tensioned wires or screws. Another option is to attach the proximal ring to a clamp in line with the tibia shaft, joined to this latter with screws (Fig. **10**) [35]. Hydroxyapatite coating improves significantly the tightness of the screws to the bone and reduces the pin tract infections [63, 64].

After the joint/epiphysis reduction, this needs to be attached to the shaft [60]. A very common circular frame scheme is based on four rings, two proximal and two distal to the main metaphyseal/shaft fracture line. First, traction is applied between the proximal and the distal holds. After this, with the help of external manoeuvres, olive wires, bended wires that become straight when tensioned, the metaphysis/diaphysis fracture reduction is obtained [60, 65, 66]. One or more intermediate rings can be helpful in reduction and in breaking the lever arm if too long [65, 66]. Some Authors advise for "lighter" constructs, characterized by only one ring at the epiphyseal site [32, 66].

Once the bone stability is reached, both at the plateau and at the tibia shaft, the ligamententous balance has to be assessed. When a clinical evident instability is present, or an epiphyseal comminution, or a vascular suture that needs to be protected, or severe soft tissue damage, or a disruption of the extensor apparatus, there is the indication for the extension of the fixator to the femur. If a mobile femur-tibial frame is planned, the hinges of the frame needs to lie along the axis of rotation of the knee. To identify the axis, a wire is inserted at the medial condyle throughout the distal femur where the centre of rotation is supposed to be. If the fluoroscopy check confirms the wire is in the right position, this would be the guide for assembling hinges [60].

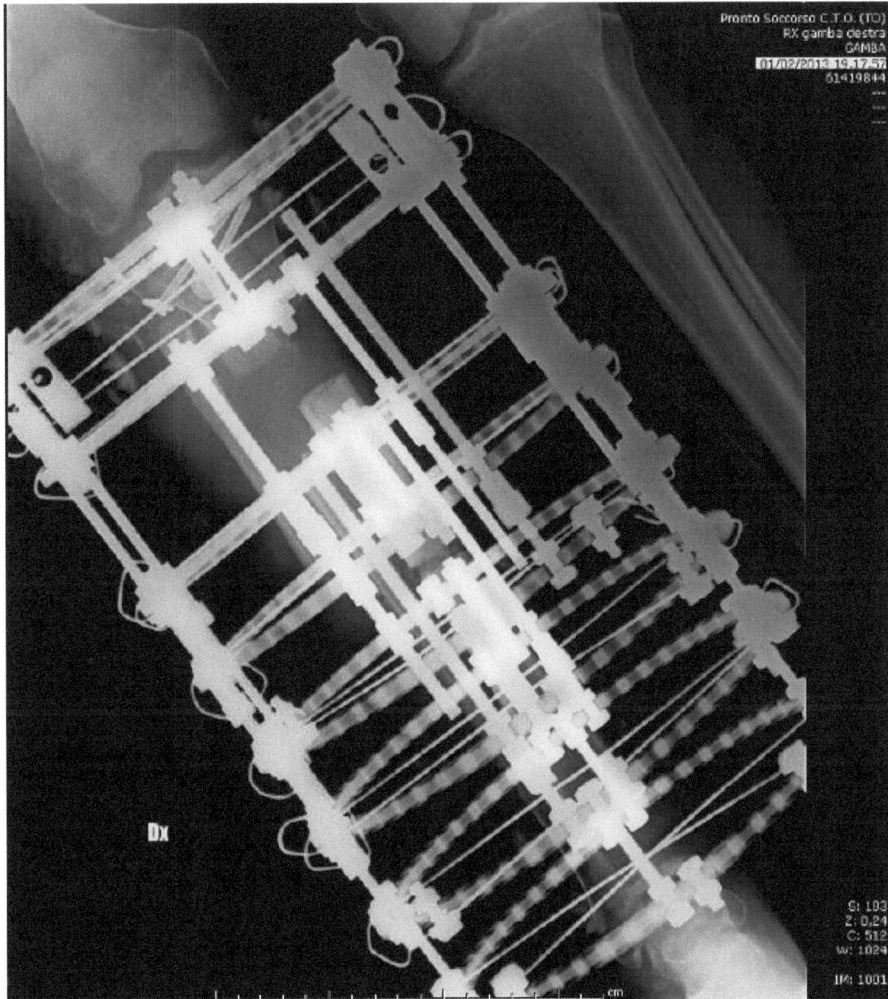

Fig. (10). Post-operative images. The traditional screw-based ORIF for the tibial plateau, double corticotomy, planned to halve the time of tibia shaft reconstruction. AP view.

A circular frame acts like a plate, allowing for some adjunctive distinctive features: it is relatively stiff at the beginning, but it changes into a more elastic device with the wires loosening during the treatment progress, it can be partially modified by operators, acting compression at the fracture site, adding or removing wires/screws, opening some nuts when more elasticity is advisable. The exclusive characteristic of the circular frame is the possibility of bone formation by means of the distractional osteogenesis: the corticotomy of the tibia shaft at a healthy site, keeping the periosteum viable, gives the possibility to transport the bone of about 1 mm per day, this way filling the gap (Figs. **10 - 15**) [67, 68].

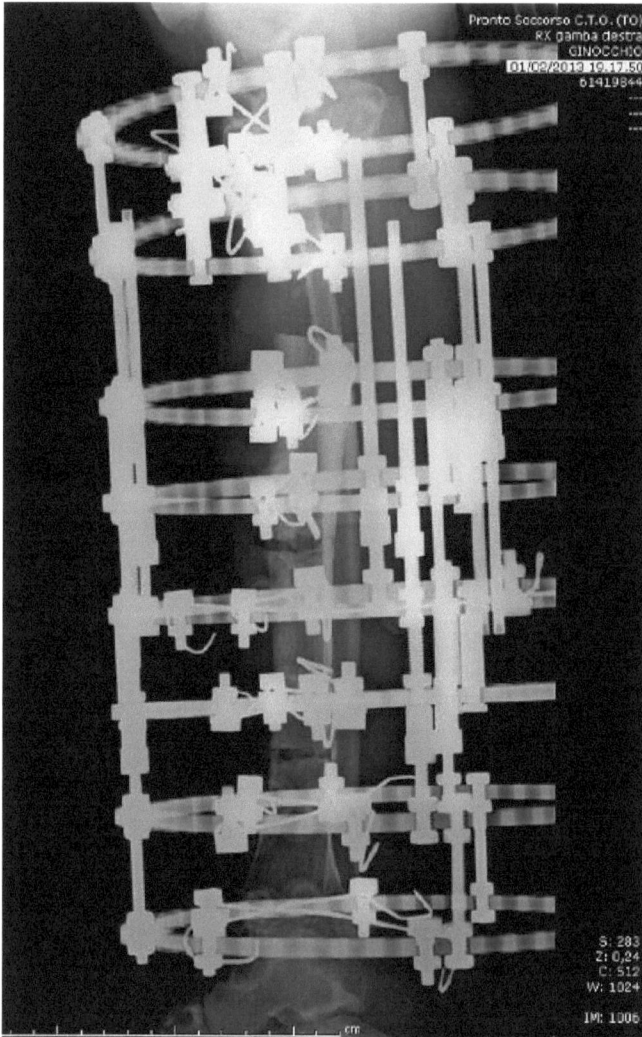

Fig. (11). Post-operative images. The traditional screw-based ORIF for the tibial plateau, double corticotomy, planned to halve the time of tibia shaft reconstruction. This treatment was performed 54 days after the trauma because of the soft tissue conditions.

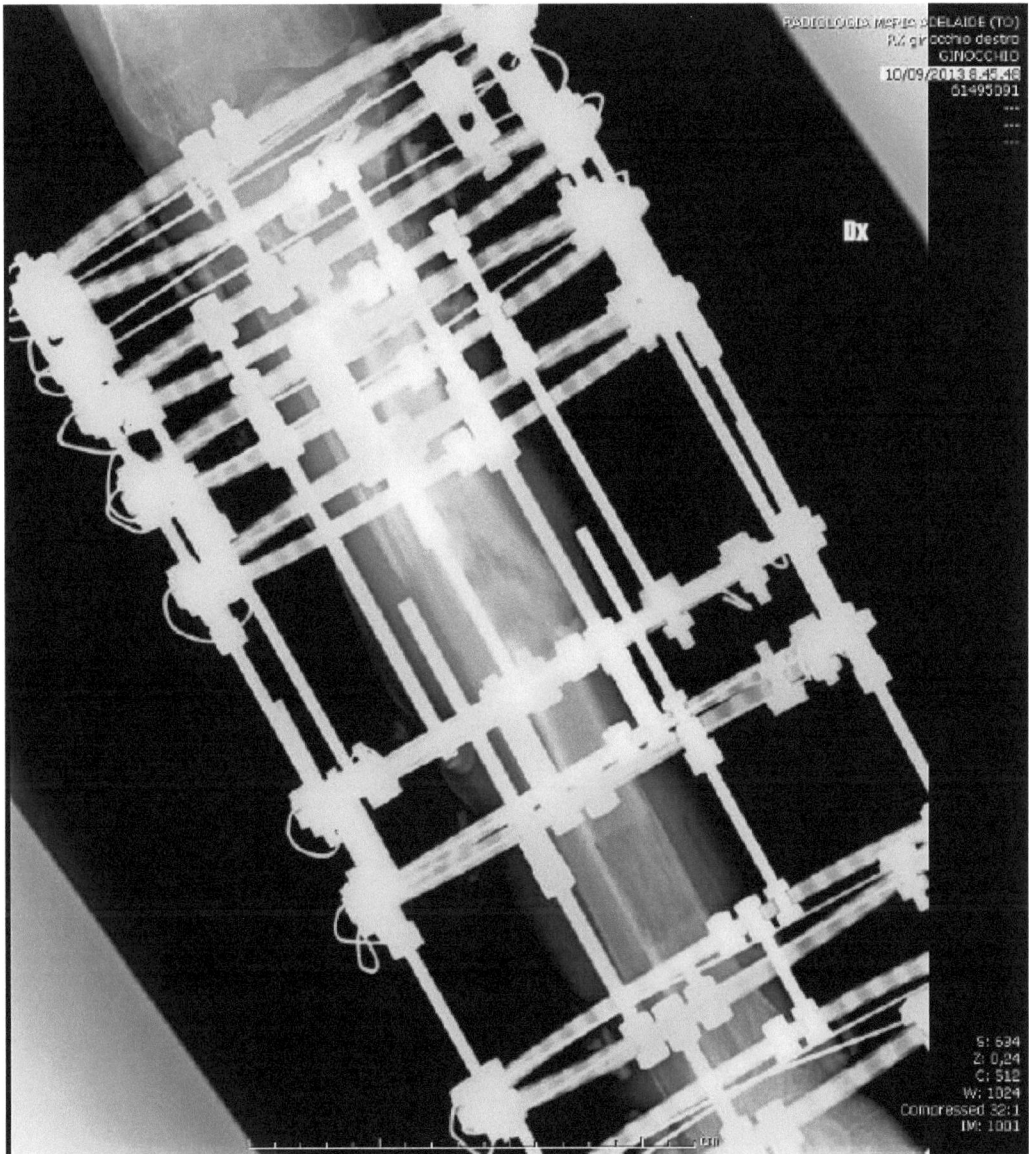

Fig. (12). September 2013: end of new bone formation and lengthening. The proximal docking point didn't reach stability.

Choosing ring diameter, the general role is to exceed the leg dimensions of at least 2 cm on every side: a safe method is to leave some more space anticipating the possible swelling [35].

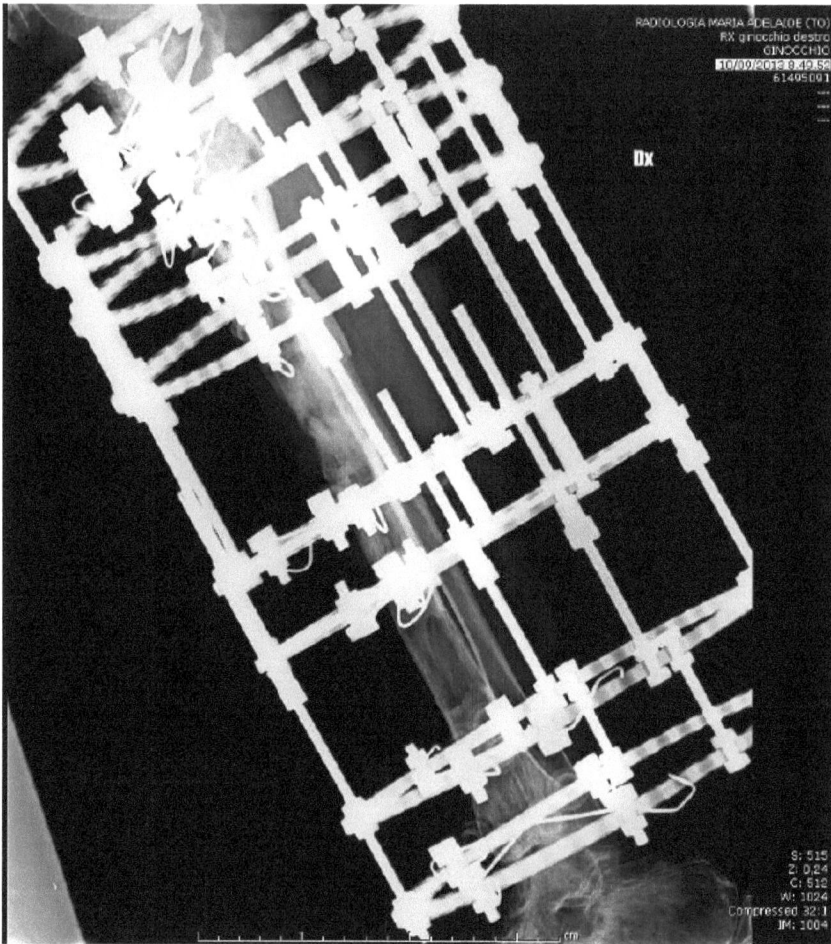

Fig. (13). September 2013: end of new bone formation and lengthening.

Even if 2/3 or 5/8 incomplete rings are available and can be helpful in allowing a wider knee range of motion (there is no impingement between the posterior section of the ring and the back side of the thigh), their use must be carefully planned, as they can collapse if the wires are over-tighten [35].

There is not a definitive indication concerning the best timing of the definitive reduction, but a prudent habit is to wait until the creases of the skin reappear because of the oedema regression and the surgical site turns into a dry and wrinkled appearance [24].

Paradoxically, a recent anatomical and clinical plate & screw-based study asserted the biological reason for an external/minimal invasive approach to the proximal tibia: the vascular pattern of the antero-lateral angiosome, where perforator branches of the anterior tibial artery are jeopardized by a traditional antero-lateral approach based on the tibialis anterior muscle (TA) detachment, makes the skin very vulnerable. A new method characterized by an L-shaped skin incision, a traditional epiphyseal and joint reduction, the TA muscle insertion to bone preserved, a fixation by means of a plate that runs under the skin but superficially to the TA fascia, with only screws crossing the muscle belly, seems to better preserve both the skin and the bone vascularization. In the clinical setting, this approach has shown to be safe and no skin necrosis or infection emerged [69]. But if a plate can safely spare the angiosome, why should not a circular external fixator do the same?

Tibial plateau fracture is a very challenging pathology. Despite an increasing amount of literature analysing the problem and which surgical strategy is the best in facing the problem, no univocal answer is on the way [70]. Even when functional results have proven to be acceptable in terms of range of movement and patient's satisfaction, a complete functional recovery is very uncommon, especially when it is considered as the comeback to sports [8, 70, 71].

In spite of this discouraging starting point, the circular external fixation has shown to be a reliable and qualified method. Functional outcome is comparable to that of ORIF, often with less complications [71 - 76].

Complications, though low rate, can be severe. Peroneal nerve is very rarely affected, but it is anyway in danger when applying the proximal wires from the lateral entrance point: if any doubt arises, a direct surgical approach could be advised [72, 77]. A thorough planning and a precise technique must be applied in reducing the tibial shaft deformity, where a varus wider than 10° is bad prognostic factor in term of post traumatic knee arthritis [72]. Pin site infections are very often reported, but this is a problem that can be easily managed in a well organized outpatient clinic.

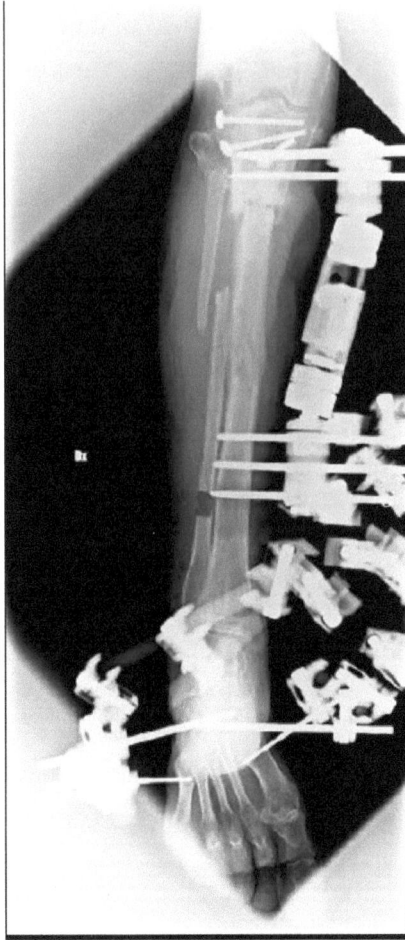

Fig. (14). The proximal docking point didn't reach stability, so in February 2014 the circular frame was removed, a new lighter monolateral frame was applied, the proximal site was stimulated by means of surgical debridement and local application of autologous bone marrow (from the iliac crest) concentrate. The monolateral frame was kept in place for 5 months.

A very important feature, that can affect the clinical results, is the psychological status of the patient: external fixation treatments are long and can be badly tolerated when the patient is not comfortable with it, when he/she does not collaborate with the surgeon, when he/she does not comply with prescriptions [78].

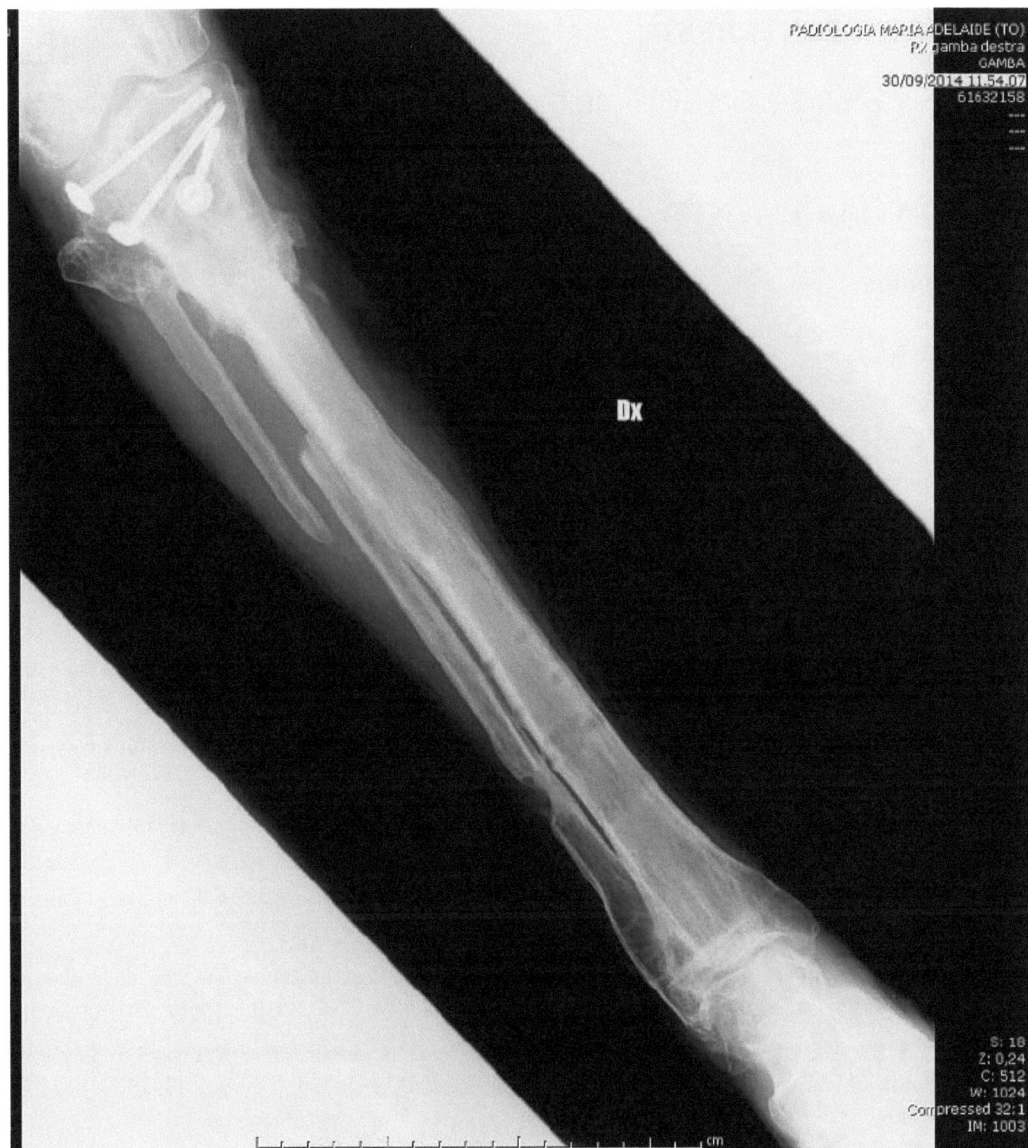

Fig. (15). Final appearance (September 2014). The Patient is not limping, the knee ROM is 0°-0°-120°, painless.

It is the author's opinion that the circular external fixation treatment for the articular fractures should be carried out in those highly qualified settings where experienced trained surgeons together with multidisciplinary (plastic and vascular surgeons, dedicated nurses, rehabilitation facilities) teams are present.

CONFLICT OF INTEREST

The author confirms that author has no conflict of interest to declare for this publication.

ACKNOWLEDGEMENTS

Declared none.

REFERENCES

[1]   Borrelli J Jr. Management of soft tissue injuries associated with tibial plateau fractures. J Knee Surg 2014; 27(1): 5-9.

[2]   Wasserstein D, Henry P, Kreder H, Paterson M, Jenkinson R. Risk factors for re-operation and mortality following the operative treatment of tibial plateau fractures in ontario, 1996-2009. J Orthop Trauma 2014. Epub ahead of print

[3]   Ariffin HM, Mahdi NM, Rhani SA, Baharudin A, Shukur MH. Modified hybrid fixator for high-energy Schatzker V and VI tibial plateau fractures. Strateg Trauma Limb Reconstr 2011; 6(1): 21-6.

[4]   Albuquerque RP, Hara R, Prado J, Schiavo L, Giordano V, do Amaral NP. Epidemiological study on tibial plateau fractures at a level I trauma center. Acta Ortop Bras 2013; 21(2): 109-15.

[5]   Levy BA, Zlowodzki MP, Graves M, Cole PA. Screening for extermity arterial injury with the arterial pressure index. Am J Emerg Med 2005; 23(5): 689-95.

[6]   Wahlquist M, Iaguilli N, Ebraheim N, Levine J. Medial tibial plateau fractures: a new classification system. J Trauma 2007; 63(6): 1418-21.

[7]   Bennett WF, Browner B. Tibial plateau fractures: a study of associated soft tissue injuries. J Orthop Trauma 1994; 8(3): 183-8.

[8]   Timmers TK, van der Ven DJ, de Vries LS, van Olden GD. Functional outcome after tibial plateau fracture osteosynthesis: a mean follow-up of 6 years. Knee 2014; 21(6): 1210-5. [Epub ahead of print].

[9]   Basques BA, Webb ML, Bohl DD, Golinvaux NS, Grauer JN. Adverse Events, Length of Stay, and Readmission Following Surgery for Tibial Plateau Fractures. J Orthop Trauma 2014; 29(3): e121-6. Epub ahead of print

[10]   Young MJ, Barrack RL. Complications of internal fixation of tibial plateau fractures. Orthop Rev 1994; 23(2): 149-54.

[11]   Lin S, Mauffrey C, Hammerberg EM, Stahel PF, Hak DJ. Surgical site infection after open reduction and internal fixation of tibial plateau fractures. Eur J Orthop Surg Traumatol 2014; 24(5): 797-803.

[12]   Colman M, Wright A, Gruen G, Siska P, Pape HC, Tarkin I. Prolonged operative time increases infection rate in tibial plateau fractures. Injury 2013; 44(2): 249-52.

[13]   Bachoura A, Guitton TG, Smith RM, Vrahas MS, Zurakowski D, Ring D. Infirmity and injury complexity are risk factors for surgical-site infection after operative fracture care. Clin Orthop Relat Res 2011; 469(9): 2621-30.

[14]   Urruela AM, Davidovitch R, Karia R, Khurana S, Egol KA. Results following operative treatment of tibial plateau fractures. J Knee Surg 2013; 26(3): 161-5.

[15]   Ruffolo MR, Gettys FK, Montijo HE, Seymour RB, Karunakar MA. Complications of high-energy bicondylar tibial plateau fractures treated with dual plating through two incisions. J Orthop Trauma 2014; 29(2): 85-90.

[16]   Pape HC, Hildebrand F, Pertschy S, *et al.* Changes in the management of femoral shaft fractures in polytrauma patients: from early total care to damage control orthopedic surgery. J Trauma 2002; 53(3): 452-61.

[17]   Pape HC, Giannoudis P, Krettek C. The timing of fracture treatment in polytrauma patients: relevance of damage control orthopedic surgery. Am J Surg 2002; 183(6): 622-9.

[18]   Giannoudis PV. Surgical priorities in damage control in polytrauma. J Bone Joint Surg Br 2003; 85(4): 478-83.

[19]   Pape HC, Grimme K, Van Griensven M, *et al.* Impact of intramedullary instrumentation *versus* damage control for femoral fractures on immunoinflammatory parameters: prospective randomized analysis by the EPOFF Study Group. J Trauma 2003; 55(1): 7-13.

[20]   Scalea TM, Boswell SA, Scott JD, Mitchell KA, Kramer ME, Pollak AN. External fixation as a bridge to intramedullary nailing for patients with multiple injuries and with femur fractures: damage control orthopedics. J Trauma 2000; 48(4): 613-21.

[21]   Harwood PJ, Giannoudis PV, van Griensven M, Krettek C, Pape HC. Alterations in the systemic inflammatory response after early total care and damage control procedures for femoral shaft fracture in severely injured patients. J Trauma 2005; 58(3): 446-52.

[22]   Rixen D, Grass G, Sauerland S, *et al.* Polytrauma Study Group of the German Trauma Society. Evaluation of criteria for temporary external fixation in risk-adapted damage control orthopedic surgery of femur shaft fractures in multiple trauma patients: "evidence-based medicine" *versus* "reality" in the trauma registry of the German Trauma Society. J Trauma 2005; 59(6): 1375-94.

[23]   Giannoudis PV, Giannoudi M, Stavlas P. Damage control orthopaedics: lessons learned. Injury 2009; 40 (Suppl. 4): S47-52.

[24]   Rüedi TP, Murphy WM, *et al.* AO Principles of Fracture Management. Stuttgart, New York 2000. 114, 499-500, 625.

[25]   Haidukewych GJ. Temporary external fixation for the management of complex intra- and periarticular fractures of the lower extremity. J Orthop Trauma 2002; 16(9): 678-85.

[26]   Egol KA, Tejwani NC, Capla EL, Wolinsky PL, Koval KJ. Staged management of high-energy proximal tibia fractures (OTA types 41): the results of a prospective, standardized protocol. J Orthop Trauma 2005; 19(7): 448-55.

[27]   Barei DP, Nork SE, Mills WJ, Henley MB, Benirschke SK. Complications associated with internal fixation of high-energy bicondylar tibial plateau fractures utilizing a two-incision technique. J Orthop Trauma 2004; 18(10): 649-57.

[28]   Anglen JO, Aleto T. Temporary transarticular external fixation of the knee and ankle. J Orthop Trauma 1998; 12(6): 431-4.

[29] Taeger G, Ruchholtz S, Waydhas C, Lewan U, Schmidt B, Nast-Kolb D. Damage control orthopedics in patients with multiple injuries is effective, time saving, and safe. J Trauma 2005; 59(2): 409-16.

[30] Sems SA, Levy BA, Dajani K, Herrera DA, Templeman DC. Incidence of deep venous thrombosis after temporary joint spanning external fixation for complex lower extremity injuries. J Trauma 2009; 66(4): 1164-6.

[31] Dirschl DR, Dawson PA. Injury severity assessment in tibial plateau fractures. Clin Orthop Relat Res 2004; (423): 85-92.

[32] Santolini F, Stella M, Chiapale D, Briano S. "Osteosintesi con fissatore esterno" in R Pessina, P Regazzoni, A Pace Le fratture dei piatti tibiali. Italy: Timeo 2011; pp. 85-97.

[33] Harwood PJ, Giannoudis PV, Probst C, Krettek C, Pape HC. The risk of local infective complications after damage control procedures for femoral shaft fracture. J Orthop Trauma 2006; 20(3): 181-9.

[34] Laible C, Earl-Royal E, Davidovitch R, Walsh M, Egol KA. Infection after spanning external fixation for high-energy tibial plateau fractures: is pin site-plate overlap a problem? J Orthop Trauma 2012; 26(2): 92-7.

[35] Santoro D, Tantavisut S, Aloj D, Karam MD. Diaphyseal osteotomy after post-traumatic malalignment. Curr Rev Musculoskelet Med 2014; 7(4): 312-22.

[36] Carroll EA, Koman LA. External fixation and temporary stabilization of femoral and tibial trauma. J Surg Orthop Adv 2011; 20(1): 74-81.

[37] Mathieu L, Bazile F, Barthélémy R, Duhamel P, Rigal S. Damage control orthopaedics in the context of battlefield injuries: the use of temporary external fixation on combat trauma soldiers. Orthop Traumatol Surg Res 2011; 97(8): 852-9.

[38] Gordon WT, Grijalva S, Potter BK. Damage control and austere environment external fixation: techniques for the civilian provider. J Surg Orthop Adv 2012; 21(1): 22-31.

[39] D'Alleyrand JC, O'Toole RV. The evolution of damage control orthopedics: current evidence and practical applications of early appropriate care. Orthop Clin North Am 2013; 44(4): 499-507.

[40] Mathieu L, Ouattara N, Poichotte A, *et al.* Temporary and definitive external fixation of war injuries: use of a French dedicated fixator. Int Orthop 2014; 38(8): 1569-76.

[41] Schatzker J, McBroom R, Bruce D. The tibial plateau fracture. The Toronto experience 1968--1975. Clin Orthop Relat Res 1979; (138): 94-104.

[42] Schatzker J. Fracture of the Tibial Plateau. In: Schatzker J, Tile M, Eds. Rationale of Operative Fracture Care. Berlin: Springer-Verlag 1988; pp. 279-95.

[43] Gustilo RB, Merkow RL, Templeman D. The management of open fractures. J Bone Joint Surg Am 1990; 72(2): 299-304.

[44] Oestern HU, Tscherne H. Pathophysiology and Classification of Soft Tissu Injuries Associated with Fractures. In: Tscherne H, Ed. Fractures with Soft Tissue Injuries. New York: Springer-Verlag 1984; pp. 1-9.

[45] Delamarter RB, Hohl M, Hopp E Jr. Ligament injuries associated with tibial plateau fractures. Clin Orthop Relat Res 1990; (250): 226-33.

[46]   Noyes FR, Barber SD, Mooar LA. A rationale for assessing sports activity levels and limitations in knee disorders. Clin Orthop Relat Res 1989; (246): 238-49.

[47]   Tegner Y, Lysholm J. Rating systems in the evaluation of knee ligament injuries. Clin Orthop Relat Res 1985; (198): 43-9.

[48]   Roos EM, Roos HP, Lohmander LS, Ekdahl C, Beynnon BD. Knee Injury and Osteoarthritis Outcome Score (KOOS)--development of a self-administered outcome measure. J Orthop Sports Phys Ther 1998; 28(2): 88-96.

[49]   Moghaddam A, Weiss S, Wölfl CG, *et al.* Cigarette smoking decreases TGF-b1 serum concentrations after long bone fracture. Injury 2010; 41(10): 1020-5.

[50]   Morris BJ, Unger RZ, Archer KR, Mathis SL, Perdue AM, Obremskey WT. Risk factors of infection after ORIF of bicondylar tibial plateau fractures. J Orthop Trauma 2013; 27(9): e196-200.

[51]   Ferreira N, Marais LC. Bicondylar tibial plateau fractures treated with fine-wire circular external fixation. Strateg Trauma Limb Reconstr 2014; 9(1): 25-32.

[52]   Narayan B, Harris C, Nayagam S. Treatment of high-energy tibial plateau fractures. Strateg Trauma Limb Reconstr 2006; 1: 18-28.

[53]   Ries MD, Meinhard BP. Medial external fixation with lateral plate internal fixation in metaphyseal tibia fractures. A report of eight cases associated with severe soft-tissue injury. Clin Orthop Relat Res 1990; (256): 215-23.

[54]   Kataria H, Sharma N, Kanojia RK. Small wire external fixation for high-energy tibial plateau fractures. J Orthop Surg (Hong Kong) 2007; 15(2): 137-43.

[55]   Ahearn N, Oppy A, Halliday R, *et al.* The outcome following fixation of bicondylar tibial plateau fractures. Bone Joint J 2014; 96-B(7): 956-62.

[56]   Barei DP, Nork SE, Mills WJ, Coles CP, Henley MB, Benirschke SK. Functional outcomes of severe bicondylar tibial plateau fractures treated with dual incisions and medial and lateral plates. J Bone Joint Surg Am 2006; 88(8): 1713-21.

[57]   Kumar A, Whittle AP. Treatment of complex (Schatzker Type VI) fractures of the tibial plateau with circular wire external fixation: retrospective case review. J Orthop Trauma 2000; 14(5): 339-44.

[58]   Ali AM, Yang L, Hashmi M, Saleh M. Bicondylar tibial plateau fractures managed with the Sheffield Hybrid Fixator Injury 2001; 32(Suppl 4)

[59]   Padanilam TG, Ebraheim NA, Frogameni A. Meniscal detachment to approach lateral tibial plateau fractures. Clin Orthop Relat Res 1995; (314): 192-8.

[60]   Katsenis D, Athanasiou V, Megas P, Tyllianakis M, Lambiris E. Minimal internal fixation augmented by small wire transfixion frames for high-energy tibial plateau fractures. J Orthop Trauma 2005; 19(4): 241-8.

[61]   Buchko GM, Johnson DH. Arthroscopy assisted operative management of tibial plateau fractures. Clin Orthop Relat Res 1996; (332): 29-36.

[62]   Reid JS, Van Slyke MA, Moulton MJ, Mann TA. Safe placement of proximal tibial transfixation wires with respect to intracapsular penetration. J Orthop Trauma 2001; 15(1): 10-7.

[63]   Magyar G, Toksvig-Larsen S, Moroni A. Hydroxyapatite coating of threaded pins enhances fixation. J Bone Joint Surg Br 1997; 79(3): 487-9.

[64]   Moroni A, Heikkila J, Magyar G, Toksvig-Larsen S, Giannini S. Fixation strength and pin tract infection of hydroxyapatite-coated tapered pins. Clin Orthop Relat Res 2001; (388): 209-17.

[65]   Bagnoli G. La metodica di Ilizarov nel trattamento delle fratture e delle pseudartrosi di gamba. Masson Italia Editori 1986; pp. 53-85.

[66]   Solomin LN. The Basic Principles of External Fixation Using the Ilizarov Device. Italy: Springer-Verlag Italia 2008; pp. 15-23. 175-177

[67]   Dagher F, Roukoz S. Compound tibial fractures with bone loss treated by the Ilizarov technique. J Bone Joint Surg Br 1991; 73(2): 316-21.

[68]   Rigal S, Merloz P, Le Nen D, Mathevon H, Masquelet AC. Bone transport techniques in posttraumatic bone defects. Orthop Traumatol Surg Res 2012; 98(1): 103-8.

[69]   Solomon LB, Boopalan PR, Chakrabarty A, Callary SA. Can tibial plateau fractures be reduced and stabilised through an angiosome-sparing antero-lateral approach? Injury 2014; 45(4): 766-74.

[70]   Ahearn N, Oppy A, Halliday R, *et al.* The outcome following fixation of bicondylar tibial plateau fractures. Bone Joint J 2014; 96-B(7): 956-62.

[71]   Hall JA, Beuerlein MJ, McKee MD. Open reduction and internal fixation compared with circular fixator application for bicondylar tibial plateau fractures. Surgical technique. J Bone Joint Surg Am 2009; 91 (Suppl. 2 Pt 1): 74-88.

[72]   Katsenis D, Dendrinos G, Kouris A, Savas N, Schoinochoritis N, Pogiatzis K. Combination of fine wire fixation and limited internal fixation for high-energy tibial plateau fractures: functional results at minimum 5-year follow-up. J Orthop Trauma 2009; 23(7): 493-501.

[73]   Mahadeva D, Costa ML, Gaffey A. Open reduction and internal fixation *versus* hybrid fixation for bicondylar/severe tibial plateau fractures: a systematic review of the literature. Arch Orthop Trauma Surg 2008; 128(10): 1169-75.

[74]   Dendrinos GK, Kontos S, Katsenis D, Dalas A. Treatment of high-energy tibial plateau fractures by the Ilizarov circular fixator. J Bone Joint Surg Br 1996; 78(5): 710-7.

[75]   Ahearn N, Oppy A, Halliday R, *et al.* The outcome following fixation of bicondylar tibial plateau fractures. Bone Joint J 2014; 96-B(7): 956-62.

[76]   Yu L, Fenglin Z. High-energy tibial plateau fractures: external fixation *versus* plate fixation. Eur J Orthop Surg Traumatol 2014; 25(3): 411-23. [Epub ahead of print].

[77]   El-Shazly M, Saleh M. Displacement of the common peroneal nerve associated with upper tibial fracture: implications for fine wire fixation. J Orthop Trauma 2002; 16(3): 204-7.

[78]   Baker MJ, Offutt SM. External fixation indications and patient selection. Clin Podiatr Med Surg 2003; 20(1): 9-26.

CHAPTER 9

Diagnosis and Treatment Strategy in Associated Lesions of Tibial Plateau Fractures

Francesco Saccia[*] and **Marco Dolfin**

Unit of Orthopaedics and Traumatology, Hospital San Giovanni Bosco, Piazza Del Donatore Del Sangue 3, 10154 Turin, Italy

Abstract: Tibial plateau fractures are associated with a broad spectrum of injuries. Associated soft tissue injuries in tibial plateau fractures can be divided as soft tissue envelope lesions, neurovascular injuries and intra-articular lesions. Careful preoperative soft tissue envelope management is important in avoiding additional injury. The neurovascular status of the extremity must be evaluated, although concomitant injuries of neurovascular structures are rare. Lesions of the ligaments and/or the menisci has been reported in several studies and may contribute, if not properly treated, to the substandard outcomes associated with this type of fractures. Traditionally, meniscal tears are reported in 20-50% cases of all the tibial plateau fractures, while ligaments lesions are reported in 10-30%. Even if the examination of knee stability and of the conditions of menisci and ligaments is not so easy, is recommended to perform a careful evaluation of the patient in order to determine associated ligamentous damage. The imaging studies routinely performed for tibial plateau fractures are plain anteroposterior and lateral radiographs and three-dimensional CT, while MRI has not yet become a standard tool. The final outcome of surgical treatment may be influenced by associated lesions of the menisci or of the knee ligaments. There is a wide uniformity of behaviours in treating meniscal tears: central tears in white zone must be resected, while peripheral lesions in red zone and meniscocapsular disjunction must be repaired. Ligamentous injuries associated with bony avulsion should be acutely treated during fracture fixation; in the absence of bony avulsion, functional and residual laxity should be addressed at a later date.

[*] **Correspondence author Francesco Saccia:** Unit of Orthopaedics and Traumatology, Hospital San Giovanni Bosco, Piazza Del Donatore Del Sangue 3, 10154 Turin, Italy; Tel: +39.011.2402439; E-mail: francesco.saccia@gmail.com

Francesco Atzori and Luigi Sabatini (Eds)

Keywords: Bony avulsion, Ligamentous injuries, Meniscal tears, Repair, Soft tissue.

INTRODUCTION

Tibial plateau fractures represent just 1% of all fractures [1 - 7], but they could have severe consequences if the broad spectrum of associated injuries is not diagnosed and treated properly. The traumatic mechanism (the amount of the force, the position of the limb during the trauma [8]) and the degree of osteopenia [9, 10] determine not only the fracture type, but the extent of soft tissue injury too. Damages of the soft tissue in tibial plateau fractures (injuries to the cruciate and collateral ligaments, the menisci, arteries and nerves) have been reported [1]. They can be divided as soft tissue envelope lesions, neurovascular injuries and intra-articular lesions. The marginal soft tissue envelope lesions affect the skin and subcutaneous tissue surrounding the proximal tibia. The neurovascular injuries affect the popliteal neurovascular bundle and the common peroneal nerve. The intra-articular lesions affect the intra-articular structures of the knee, basically menisci and ligaments. They are the most frequent associated lesions in tibial plateau fractures.

SOFT TISSUE ENVELOPE LESIONS AND NEUROVASCULAR INJURIES

To achieve a good outcome in complex tibial plateau fracture it is mandatory to evaluate and correctly treat any associated soft tissue lesion. This tissues are often involved in high-energy knee trauma because of the thickness of subcutaneous tissue, making it vulnerable both from the inside (displacement of bone fragments) and from the outside (direct external forces). Involvement of soft tissues around the knee increases the risk of complications following the treatment of high-energy knee trauma [11]. The physical examination should always include a thorough assessment of the soft tissue envelope. In fact, an high energy trauma should cause cutaneous and subcutaneous damage, venous and nervous compromise, increasing the risk of early and late complications [11, 13, 14]. Severe soft tissue injuries may not allow primary plating of the fracture, requiring instead the use of a spanning external fixator [12]. In the case of an open fracture, when the soft tissue envelope is completely disrupted, cleansing of the open wound is required, followed by a complete coverage of the bone segment of the tibia, reducing future risks of infection [13]. The acute treatment of soft tissue injuries consists in reducing as much as possible the inflammatory response, using NSAIDs and cryotherapy, and immobilizing the knee using splints, transkeletal traction or external fixators [15 - 17, 19]. Splints are usually used in fractures without a severe soft tissue impairment, because they require a circumferential dressing that reduce the possibility of a constant evaluation of the skin. In high energy trauma it is preferable to use a transkeletal traction or a temporary knee-spanning external fixator, with the aim of achieving a fracture reduction by the process of ligamentotaxis [11] (Fig. **1a-b**) .

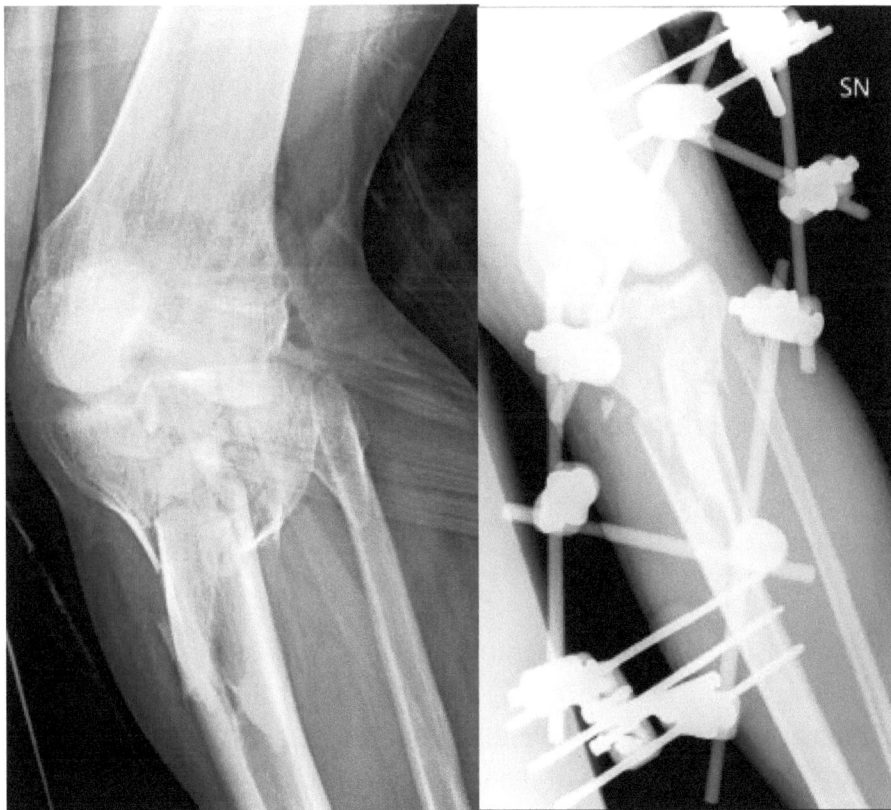

Fig. (1). Temporary placement of knee-spanning external-fixator for a Schatzker VI tibial plateau fracture in a high-energy trauma.

The neurovascular status of the extremity must be carefully evaluated, although concomitant injuries of neurovascular structures are rare in association with tibial plateau fractures. The possibility of vascular injury occurs in about 2% [20, 21] of bicondylar tibial plateau fractures (Schatzker V and Schatzker VI types). Evaluation and palpation of the peripheral pulses must be performed; if there is an abnormality on palpation pulses, a vascular consult may be needed [22]. An ankle-brachial index of the extremity less than 0.9 indicates that vascular injury is very likely [12]. Use of arteriography or of a CT angiography is recommended when there is an alteration of the arterial pulse or a strong suspicion of arterial injury, or even in associated compartment syndrome. When the energy of the trauma is likely to cause a knee dislocation or a Schatzker type IV, V or VI fracture, the execution of a CT angiography should be considered. Multi-slice CT angiography is a reliable, sensitive and specific non-invasive imaging modality for arterial evaluation in this type of fracture [23]. Ultrasound evaluation has not the same sensibility and specificity in detecting intimal arterial damage, so it cannot be considered as a viable alternative to arteriography [6]. Impaired sensorimotor status may indicate compartment syndrome; impaired dorsal flexion may indicate peroneal nerve injury [12]. The strength of dorsiflexion and eversion will help evaluate the peroneal nerve. It is important to examine and document peroneal nerve function before surgery because of the possibility of a stretch injury: motor and sensory function of the nerve proximal and distal to the injury should be assessed [22]. The frequency of injuries to the peroneal nerve or of an involvement of the popliteal vessels is higher if the lateral collateral ligament complex is disrupted [6].

INTRA-ARTICULAR ASSOCIATED LESIONS

With the increasing use of pre-operative MRI, the incidence of associated intra-articular lesions seems to be even higher than previously thought [24, 25]. It is often difficult to perform a complete and thorough clinical examination of knee stability and associated lesions of the soft tissue structures. This should lead to an incomplete diagnosis of the conditions of menisci and ligaments. The underestimation of associated injuries is one of the responsible of an insufficient treatment, causing an insufficient long-term result [26]. The treatment of intra-articular associated lesions is still debated. Talking about ligament injuries, it is well known that some these (*e.g.* medial collateral ligament tear) heal spontaneously with nonoperative care and good clinical outcome. However, a wide spectrum of other injuries (anterior or posterior cruciate ligament tears or multiligament knee injuries) has better functional results if treated surgically, as reported in literature [26].

Epidemiology

As previously stated, the incidence of intra-articular lesions associated to tibial plateau fractures is higher than thought in the past years, when pre-operative MRI of the knee was not widely performed. Traditionally, meniscal tears in association with tibial plateau fractures are reported in 20-50% cases, while ligaments lesions are reported in 10-30% cases [27].

Colletti *et al.* analyzed retrospectively 29 MRI scans of 29 patients with acute tibial plateau fractures, reporting that "the three most common associated injuries were MCL injuries (55% of patients), lateral meniscus tears (45%) and ACL injuries (41%). Anterior cruciate ligament injuries were associated with lateral meniscus tears in 75%" [28].

Shepherd *et al.* performed an MRI in 20 consecutive nonoperative tibial plateau fractures: in 18 patients MRI showed injuries to the soft tissues. 16 of them had a meniscal tear, while 8 patients of this 18 had a complete ligament tear [29].

Asik *et al.* reviewed retrospectively the effectiveness of arthroscopy assisted surgery in the treatment of 45 closed tibial plateau fractures. They noted an MCL injury in 39% of patients, an LCL injury in 10%, an ACL injury in 6%, a medial meniscus tear in 17% and a lateral meniscus tear in 33%. The tibial intercondylar eminence was avulsed in 7% of fractures [30].

Gardner *et al.* performed a prospective cohort study on 103 patients with operative tibial plateau fractures. Soft tissue injuries were assessed by MRI. The overall incidence of injury to soft tissues was very high, with only one patient (1%) without any soft tissue injury. "Seventy-nine patients (77%) sustained a lesion of 1 or more cruciate or collateral ligaments. Ninety-four patients (91%) had evidence of lateral meniscus pathology. Forty-five patients (44%) had medial meniscus tears. Seventy patients(68%) had tears of 1 or more of the posterolateral corner structures of the knee" [31].

Abdel-Hamid *et al.* published a retrospective analysis of 98 cases of tibial plateau fractures which underwent to arthroscopic evaluation of soft tissue injuries. They found that the higher soft tissue injury rate is represented in Schatzker type II fracture, which is also the most frequent type of fracture. 56 (57%) of the 98 tibial plateau fractures evaluated in this study had also a meniscal tear (the most common associated soft tissue injury) on the same side. The presence of a meniscal tear is not significantly correlated with the type of fracture. The area of the meniscus most frequently affected is the peripheral one, much more than the central one with radial or flap tears. ACL injury represents the second most common associated lesion, found in 24 of these 98 cases (25%), divided into tibial avulsion, partial tear and midsubstance rupture. ACL injury occurs more frequently in type IV and type VI fractures. In a few cases were found other ligament injury (PCL in 5 cases, MCL in 3 cases, LCL in 3 cases) [1].

Mustonen *et al.* reported "abnormal menisci detectable with MRI in 24 on 39 patients with tibial plateau fractures, for a total of 33 abnormal menisci (42%). The meniscal abnormalities were 17 contusions (52%), 11 longitudinal tears (33%), six horizontal tears (18%), six radial tears (18%) and four flap tears (12%). A stable meniscal tear was found in only 2 of the 16 tibial plateau fractures with an associated meniscal lesion. There were no significant correlation between degree of articular depression and site or morphologic features of the meniscal injury. No significant correlation was found between Schatzker type of fracture and meniscal findings." They concluded that an unstable meniscal lesion could be found in about 1/3 of this fractures, and that if a meniscal injury is found preoperatively, the treatment of the meniscal tear should be performed during the time of fracture fixation, avoiding a two-stage procedure [32].

Chan *et al.*, in a series of 54 patients who received arthroscopy -assisted surgery for tibial plateau fractures, reported that 35 of them (65%) had associated intra-articular lesions. Among these 35 patients, meniscal tear was noted in 21 knees. There were 3 medial and 19 lateral meniscal injuries. One knee had both medial and lateral meniscal pathology. Ligament injuries were noted in 22 knees with 24 lesions including 11 ACL avulsion fractures, 3 ACL partial ruptures, 5 PCL partial ruptures, 2 MCL partial ruptures, and 3 LCL avulsions in their insertion on the fibula. There were 2 combined ligament injuries (ACL and MCL partial rupture in 1 and ACL and LCL avulsion fracture in 1) [7].

Stannard *et al.* documented the incidence and the pattern of meniscal and ligament injuries occurred in 103 patients with fractures of the tibial plateau after an high-energy trauma. Analyzing MRI scans, at least one ligament torn was found in 73 patients and in 53 of them the injury was extended to other ligaments. Knee dislocation occurred in twenty-seven patients, with the complete tear of central pivot. 60 meniscus tears were found in fifty (49%) patients. "25 of this 60 lesions were found in the medial meniscus and 35 in the lateral meniscus. In ten patients the lesion was found both in the medial and in the lateral meniscus" [26].

Urruela *et al.* reported that in 57% (55) of 94 patients (2 of them with a bilateral tibial plateau fracture) there were significant associated intra-articular soft tissue injuries: 49 lateral and 6 medial meniscus tears [33].

In a retrospective study, Spiro *et al.* reviewed 54 consecutive patients with tibial plateau fractures. They stated that 82 % of the patients had accompanying soft-tissue injuries, including 46.3 % with meniscal tears (lateral meniscus tear = 35.2 %; medial meniscus tear = 11.1 %), 59.3 % with collateral ligament lesions, 44.5 % with cruciate ligament lesions and 14.8 % with patellar retinaculum lesions. Multiple soft- tissue injuries were seen in 54.0 % of the fractures [34]. Recently, Chen *et al.* performed a systematic review of the literature "to summarize the recent clinical outcomes of patients undergoing arthroscopy-assisted reduction and internal fixation (ARIF) for tibial plateau fractures. The search criteria initially identified 141 articles, and 19 studies were included in this systematic review. There were 2 retrospective comparative studies, 16 case series studies, and one clinical series based on a technique note. There were a total of 609 patients in this systematic review, with a mean follow-up time of 52.5 months". Concomitant injuries were common: meniscus and ACL injuries were the most common combined soft tissue injuries reported in 18 of 19 studies. A total of 236 patients (42.2%) also had meniscal injuries and 119 patients (21.3%) also had ACL injuries [2]. To summarize the literature's data, an associated intra-articular lesion must be expected in more than 50% of tibial plateau fractures, tears of lateral meniscus being the most frequent lesion, followed by ACL and MCL injuries.

DIAGNOSIS

Clinical Evaluation

Examination of knee stability and of the status of menisci and ligaments is often difficult because of pain and hemarthrosis (when the articular capsule is not been disrupted). The description of injury mechanism can be helpful to suspect the pattern of meniscal and ligamentous injuries. External forces that can cause a tibial plateau fracure may be directed medially, laterally, or axially. An example of a valgus force moment are often classic "bumper fractures", caused by motor vehicle *versus* pedestrian accidents. In other cases, the traumatic mechanism is "a combination of both axial and varus or valgus directed forces, where the femoral condyles act as an anvil imparting a combination of both shearing and compressive force to the underlying tibial plateau" [6]. It is often difficult to understand the precise type of the traumatic mechanism. However, "it is useful to ascertain the level of force involved in the injury, specifically high-energy or low-energy forces" [35], to evaluate the risk of associated lesions. During the clinical examination it is important to evaluate the limitation of the active and passive range of motion, due to pain, swelling and a muscle guarding or spasm, that make it difficult to assess the real extent of the injury. In all cases, especially after high energy trauma, a complete vascular and neurologic evaluation of the injured extremity should be performed [6,   35]. In case of tense hemarthrosis, arthrocentesis could reduce pain and facilitate the physical assessment of ligaments and menisci. Anyway, in the great majority of patients, the physical evaluation of knee stability is too painful, so the ligaments should be tested under anesthesia. Moreover, it is difficult to state if instability is due to ligamentous instability or articular depression.

Imaging

The imaging studies routinely performed for tibial plateau fractures are plain anteroposterior (AP) and lateral radiographs centered on the knee, with the AP view angle 10 degrees in a craniocaudal direction to approximate the posterior slope of the tibial plateau, and three-dimensional CT, which is the standard tool in analyzing tibial plateau fractures and the main tool to perform an adequate pre-operative planning. Although MRI evaluates both osseous and soft tissue injuries, it has not yet become a standard tool in analyzing tibial plateau fractures, even if it is largely considered the gold standard in identifying meniscal and ligamentous injuries. The routinely use of MRI in tibial plateau fractures is still debated. The advent and spreading of ARIF (arthroscopic reduction and internal fixation) for Schatzker type I, II and III and arthroscopic-assisted ORIF (open reduction and internal fixation) in other types (despite a higher risk of compartment syndrome for fluid extravasation from the fracture [36]) has made easier the intra-operative detection of meniscal and cruciate ligament injuries. Collateral ligaments injuries, which are not clearly and entirely detectable with the sole artrhroscopy, are anyway usually left untreated in the acute setting, with the exception of osseous avulsions, so their immediate diagnosis can be considered not paramount. However, severe articles have been written which address the utility of MRI in the detection of intra- articular lesions associated to tibial plateau fractures.

Colletti *et al.* conducted a retrospective study on MRI examinations performed on 29 patients with acute tibial plateau fractures. They concluded that "MR imaging can provide precise anatomic detail of tibial plateau fracture patterns and their severity along with the simultaneous evaluation of extraosseous structures" [28].

Fischbach *et al.* compared MRI and CT in assessing the type of fracture, degree of comminution and amount of articular surface depression in acute tibial plateau fractures and in describing the associated soft tissue injuries in 29 consecutive patients. They concluded that "MRI allows a detailed assessment of acute tibial plateau fractures and can replace conventional CT, and that the high rate of fracture- associated soft tissue lesions makes MRI an especially valuable tool" [37].

Asik *et al.* reviewed retrospectively the effectiveness of arthroscopy assisted surgery in the treatment of 45 closed tibial plateau fractures. "4P (anteroposterior, lateral and oblique) radiography were obtained in all patients preoperatively. Computed tomography (CT) with three- dimensional reconstruction was performed in 26 patients and magnetic resonance imaging was performed in just 8 patients" [30].

Shepherd *et al.* performed an MRI to register the incidence of meniscus and ligament tears in 20 consecutive undisplaced and minimally displaced tibial plateau fractures which would have been otherwise amenable to nonoperative management: in 18 cases MRI showed significant injuries to the soft tissues [29].

Gardner *et al.* performed a prospective cohort study on 103 patients with operative tibial plateau fractures. All patients were assessed with standard x-ray examinations and subsequently an MRI. The overall incidence of injury to soft tissues was very high, with only one patient (1%) in the series with complete absence of any soft tissue injury.

They concluded that the incidence of complete ligamentous or meniscal disruption associated with operative tibial plateau fractures was higher than previously reported, and even though the clinical significance of injury of these structures is unknown, the treating surgeon should be aware that a variety of soft tissue injuries are common in these fractures. In addition, all fractures had at least 1 cortical split visible on magnetic resonance imaging, implying that pure depression patterns are very rare or may not exist [25].

Mui *et al.* compared "CT and MRI in patients with tibial plateau fracture, to understand the real accuracy of CT in the evaluation of ligament tears and avulsions in these patients and to evaluate if the presence of a meniscal injury is directly correlated to the presence or severity of fracture gap and articular depression. CT registered 80% sensitivity and 98% specificity with torn ligaments".

Although the degree of fracture gap and articular depression was significantly greater in patients with meniscal injury compared with those without meniscal injury, no direct correlation has been demonstrated to predict with a good degree of sensitivity and specificity the presence of meniscal lesions in different types of fracture. Authors concluded that immediately after the trauma, CT offers high sensitivity and specificity for showing osseous avulsions, and a high negative predictive value for excluding ligament injury.

MRI keeps a fundamental role in detecting a meniscal injury before surgery [38].

Mustonen *et al.* evaluated "the prevalence of unstable meniscal tears in tibial plateau fractures, cataloging type and location of meniscal injuries found as associated lesions. 39 patients (78 menisci) undergone knee CT and MRI. They found an unstable tear in 14 of the 16 patients with a meniscal tear, without any significant correlation between degree of articular depression and site or morphologic features of the meniscal injury. The same lack of statistical correlation was found between normal menisci and degree of articular depression, nor was a significant correlation found between differing fracture groups and meniscal findings. They concluded that in tibial plateau fractures there is a high prevalence (36% of patients) of unstable meniscal tears"; that's why it is essential to make an accurate diagnosis before surgery, to have the opportunity to treat this type of injury intraoperatively [32].

Stannard *et al.* reported the incidence and the pattern of meniscal and ligament injuries occurred in "103 patients with tibial plateau fracture after a high-energy trauma. 71% patients had at least one ligament torn on MRI scans, 53% patients had multiple ligament injuries. 49% patients sustained 60 meniscus tears". To reduce the risk of underestimation of this associated lesions, they developed a treatment protocol including a preoperative MRI on these patients [26].

On the contrary, many literature have been published about the possibility to detect intra-articular associated lesions basing on radiographic signs or CT-scan measurements.

Gardner *et al.* evaluated 62 patients with Schatzker type II fractures, measuring the degree of fracture depression and condylar widening on anteroposterior (AP) plain radiographs. They wanted to know if there could be a significant correlation between these data and the presence of soft tissue associated lesions on MRI. "When depression was greater than 6 mm and widening was greater than 5 mm, lateral meniscal injury occurred in 83% of fractures, compared with 50% of fractures with less displacement. When either depression or widening was at least 8 mm, medial meniscal injury occurred more frequently (depression 53%, widening 78%, *versus* neither 15%). If the displacement is minimum (<4 mm) no

LCL and PCL tears were found, but the incidence of injury raised to 30% with increasing displacement. They concluded that due to the limited availability of MRI in some centers, these two measures should be considered in planning open or arthroscopic treatment methods for soft-tissue associated lesions" [39].

Abdel-Hamid *et al.* performed a retrospective analysis of 98 cases of tibial plateau fractures which underwent to arthroscopic evaluation of soft tissue injuries. All patients underwent anteroposterior and lateral plain radiography and CT scanning of their injured knees, while MRI was never performed and the soft tissue injuries evaluation was exclusively arthroscopic [1].

Chan *et al.*, reported that 35 of 54 (65%) patients who received arthroscopy - assisted surgery for tibial plateau fractures had associated intra-articular lesions. All patients underwent plain film study in anteroposterior and lateral views as well as computed tomography of each knee, while MRI was never performed [7].

Ringus *et al.* performed a study "to determine if the degree of lateral tibial plateau fracture depression on CT images predicted the presence of lateral meniscus tears. Degree of plateau depression was measured in millimeters by CT. Operative reports were retrospectively reviewed to determine if the lateral meniscus tear was intact or torn at the time of surgery. Twenty-eight patients had a lateral meniscus tear noted at the time of surgery. Patients with > or =10 mm of plateau depression had an eight-fold increase in risk of having a lateral meniscus tear compared to those with <10 mm of depression. This study demonstrated an association between the amount of tibial plateau depression and the likelihood of a lateral meniscus tear" [40].

As Gardner *et al.* previously, Durakbasa *et al.* published a study which had the purpose to determine the plain radiographic signs that can be indicative of meniscal injuries in Schatzker type II tibial plateau fractures. The lateral plateau depression and lateral plateau widening were measured on anteroposterior knee radiographs in 20 patients with Schatzker type II tibial plateau fracture.

Meniscal injury was present in 12 patients. The lateral plateau depression and lateral plateau widening measurements were compared between those who had meniscal injury and those who did not. They concluded that "a plain anteroposterior radiograph depicting a lateral plateau depression = 14 mm and/or a lateral plateau widening =10 mm is associated with a significantly increased risk of meniscal injury in Schatzker type II tibial plateau fractures" [41].

With the same purpose, Spiro *et al.* reviewed 54 consecutive patients with tibial plateau fractures. The amount of articular depression was assessed from MDCT scans. They searched for ligamentous and meniscal injuries on MRI images. Their conclusions were that "articular depression is a potential predictor of specific meniscal and ligamentous injuries in acute tibial plateau fracture.

However, an MRI evaluation is recommended with respect to associated soft-tissue injuries, especially when the CT scan reveals a severe depression of the tibial plateau" [34].

TREATMENT STRATEGY

The goals in the surgical treatment of tibial plateau fractures are restoration of articular surface, axis, meniscal integrity, and stability, to obtain painless motion and knee stability and avoid or postpone posttraumatic arthritis. Associated lesions of the menisci or of the knee ligaments can influence the final outcome. Non-anatomic reduction of the joint surface, malalignment, and unaddressed associated soft- tissue lesions may promote the onset of post-traumatic arthritis in these patients [34]. Inappropriate treatment of the soft tissue injuries would have a negative influence on long-term clinical results [2, 5, 7]. The extent of associated lesions is different and sometimes can affect in an important way the final outcome; the treatment of these injuries during fracture fixation is not always so easy [1]. "The use of arthroscopy in the treatment of tibial plateau fractures facilitates a more accurate diagnosis of associated lesions. Although the treatment of these lesions is not always surgical, their presence can influence the post-operative rehabilitation and may delay the return to activities of daily living, work and sport. Although a good osteosynthesis under fluoroscopic control allows good results, the fact of not having a direct arthroscopic control is likely to underestimate the associated lesions" [42]. ARIF advantages are represented by "a better exposure of the articular surface, evacuation of hemarthrosis and chondral debris, decreased morbidity, shorter hospital stay, the possibility to confirm the diagnosis and immediately treat associated intra-articular injuries, eliminating a major cause of secondary procedures and poor results" [43].

Meniscal Tears: Timing, Treatment and Post-Operative Care

Even though the treatment of intra-articular lesions associated to tibial plateau fractures is still debated, there is a wide uniformity of behaviours in treating meniscal lesions. Basically, central tears in white zone must be resected, leaving as much meniscal tissue as possible, while peripheral lesions in red zone and meniscocapsular disjunction must be repaired. Unstable meniscal tears can lead to pain and locking of the knee. In addition, patients may benefit from the chondroprotective effect of an intact meniscus.

At a mean follow-up of 7.6 years after ORIF for tibial plateau fractures, Honkonen found that 44% of the patients had secondary osteoarthritis, and 74% of these patients had undergone meniscectomy [2, 44]. While there is no agreement on correct timing of surgical treatment for ligamentous injuries, is universally accepted that meniscal tears must be treated contextually to fracture reduction and fixation. One of the main advantages of ARIF and artrhoscopy assisted surgery *versus* ORIF is the possibility to visualize and treat every meniscal tear without the need of capsulotomy, another advantage is the possibility to visualize the entire articular surface without need for meniscal detachment and repair as compared with open treatment requiring arthrotomy.

Some authors, like Abdel-Hamid *et al.*, perform meniscal treatment before fracture fixation because of an easier access to the meniscus due to the fracture [1], but the meniscal repair can be performed after fracture reduction and fixation too. Multiple patterns of meniscal tears have been detected in association with tibial plateau fractures.

Durakbasa *et al.*, in their study which had the purpose to determine the plain radiographic signs that can be indicative of meniscal injuries in Schatzker type II tibial plateau fractures, detected 12 lateral meniscal tears in 20 patients. There were three vertical tears and nine peripheral meniscal detachments [41].

Mustonen *et al.* evaluated "the prevalence, type, and location of meniscal injuries to assess the prevalence of unstable meniscal tears in tibial plateau fractures. In 24 of the 39 patients in this study were found abnormal menisci, for a total of 33 abnormal menisci (42%). The abnormalities detected are divided into 11 vertical tears (33%), 17 contusions (52%), four flap tears (12%), six horizontal tears (18%), and six radial tears (18%). Among the 16 patients with meniscal tears (41% of the 39), 14 patients had an unstable tear" [32].

In their retrospective study performed on 29 MRI scans of 29 patients with acute tibial plateau fractures, Colletti *et al.* noted a lateral meniscus tear in 45% of patients and a medial meniscus tear in 21% of patients [28].

In a case series of 18 consecutive patients with complex tibial plateau fractures, Chan *et al.* found "a rupture or detachment of the meniscus in 61% of patients (11 knees). There was a medial meniscus lesion in 2 knees, a lateral meniscus lesion in 7 knees, and in 2 knees they found a lesion in both the menisci. A meniscal suture was performed in eleven cases, a partial resection in 2 cases. No total meniscectomy was performed in this series. Meniscal tears were considered for repair if located within 5 mm of the meniscosynovial junction" [45].

In 98 cases of tibial plateau fractures which underwent to arthroscopic evaluation of soft tissue injuries, Abdel-Hamid *et al.* noted a meniscal tear in 56 patients (57%). These injuries always occurred on the same side as the fracture. It was not found a direct correlation between fracture type and incidence of meniscal tears. In most cases the meniscal injury is a peripheral tear, significantly more frequent than radial or flap tears. They reported 37 (38%) peripheral tears, which were treated with arthroscopic inside-out suture repair, 18 (18%) radial tears and 1 (1%) flap tear, all treated with partial meniscectomy [1].

Chan *et al.*, in a series of 54 patients who received arthroscopy -assisted surgery for tibial plateau fractures, reported a meniscal lesion in 21 knees. There were 3 medial and 19 lateral meniscal injuries. One knee had both medial and lateral meniscus tears. A meniscal suture was performed on fifteen menisci, a partial resection in seven, and none of the menisci was totally removed. The treatment of associated lesions was performed only after "a complete fracture fixation. Meniscal tears were repaired regardless of patient age because of the likelihood of healing, only when they were within 5 mm of the meniscosynovial junction. Of the various techniques for meniscal repair, the authors favored the inside- out technique using meniscal repair cannulas for middle one-third to posterior one-third horn tears and the outside-in technique for anterior one third horn tears" [7]. Ruiz-Iban *et al.* reviewed "15 cases of repaired meniscal tears in 14 patients, in a cohort of 51 tibial plateau fractures treated with ARIF. There were 14 injuries of the lateral meniscus and 1 longitudinal peripheral tear of the medial meniscus. Techniques used were an outside-in technique for the anterior horn and all-inside repair for the body and posterior horn lesions. Patients were followed for a mean (SD) of 4.83 (1.01) years. The mean (SD) Lysholm score was 88.6 (12.4). The mean (SD) IKDC score was 79.3 (19.3). There was a small decrease of the activity level according to the Tegner score when compared with the preoperative situation (1.20 [1.82], P = .022). They were asymptomatic in all the cases. 12 of 13 meniscal lesions had healed completely, as seen with a second look-arthroscopy, and a radial tear had healed partially in the vascular zone. In one of the cases that healed in the previous site of lesion, a new tear was found in a different location". They concluded that "meniscal repair of tears associated with tibial plateau fractures has good results, as second-look arthroscopy confirmed complete healing in 92% of meniscal tears when performed" [46].

Forman *et al.* performed a study with the purpose to determine what patient and injury factors are associated with the presence of a meniscus tear in tibial plateau fractures. They also sought to compare functional outcome, pain scores, and range of motion between patient groups with and without meniscal injury. A total of 99 patients with 101 acute tibial plateau fractures were included in the study cohort. Patients were divided into two groups: those with and without meniscus tears at the time of initial injury. They found that degree of tibial plateau depression was the only significant predictor of meniscal injury. They also found no significant difference in the functional outcome, pain scores, and knee range of motion between the group with and without meniscus tears at the longest follow-up interval. They concluded that these findings suggest that acute repair of meniscal injury following traumatic fracture of the tibial plateau could produce functional results similar to those patients that did not sustain a meniscus tear [47].

Chen *et al.* recently published a systematic review of the literature: meniscal tears could be noted in 42.2% of all tibial plateau fractures of the 609 patients in the 19 studies which matched the inclusion criteria. The most common types of meniscal tears were peripheral tears and radial tears. They stated that meniscal repair of meniscus tears associated to tibial plateau fractures should be performed whenever possible, and that the high healing rate of meniscal repair is pretty encouraging, and it may be attributed to several causes, such as acute repair, a conservative postoperative protocol, and the local environment with easy access to the bone marrow [2].

In conclusion, as stated by the literature, all meniscal tears associated to tibial plateau fractures must be treated contextually to the fixation of the fracture.

Meniscal repair must be performed whenever possible, but reserved to meniscus tears located within 5 mm of the meniscosynovial junction, which have a high healing rate.

Inside-out, outside-in and all-inside techniques can be used, usually with a preference for inside-out and all-inside techniques for the body and the posterior horn of the meniscus, while choosing the outside-in technique for the anterior horn. "The fibrous tissue must be removed, the walls of the tear must be debrided using a basket punch, a rasp or a shaver.

Freshening must essentially be done on the outer part of the meniscus in order to promote the healing response and to preserve meniscal tissue in the inner part. In some cases, multiple perforations can be made with a needle in the meniscal rim to stimulate the bleeding through vascular channels. Whatever the devices and the location of the meniscal tear, the implants or the sutures are routinely inserted through the ipsilateral portal for the posterior segment and the contralateral portal for the middle segment, placing a number of sutures sufficient to avoid gaps of more than 3-5 mm. Sutures must be nonabsorbable or slowly absorbable" [48]. Outside-in repair is particularly well-suited for anterior horn tears that cannot be approached from a desirable angle with all-inside or inside-out technique. The technique is easy and can be performed with 2 18-gauge spinal needles, a suture grasper, and nonabsorbable suture. However, far posterior horn tears that approach the midline are difficult to safely access, due to the danger of injury to the neurovascular structures with spinal needle placement.

Inside-out repair is considered the historical "gold standard" of meniscal repair techniques. It allows repair of extensive tears that would otherwise require both anterior and posterior approaches with outside-in techniques, and it allows for biomechanically favorable, vertical mattress suture configuration. However, the approach is difficult for far posterior horn tears that approach the midline, due to the risk of neurovascular injury with needle passage, and this technique is difficult for anterior zone tears, due to suboptimal trajectory afforded by portals and rigid cannulas. Moreover, it requires open posterolateral or posteromedial exposure.

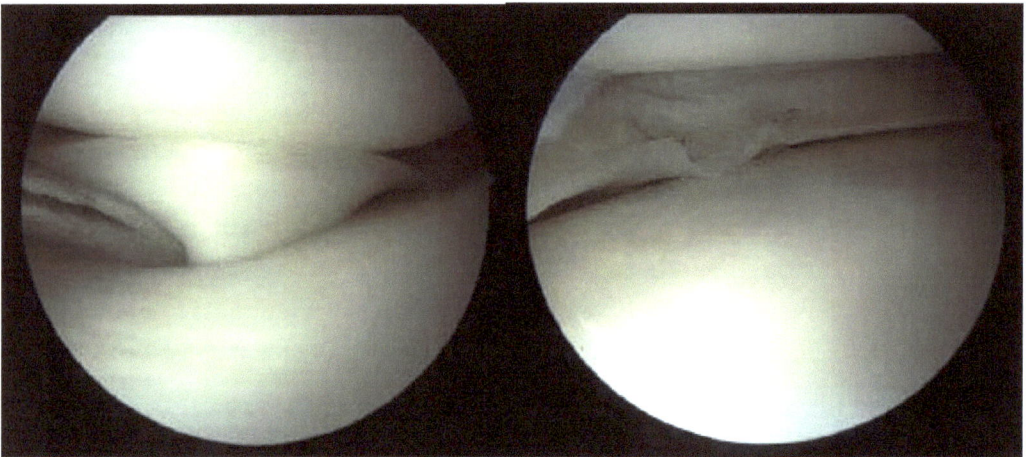

Fig. (2). All-inside repair is a particularly useful for repairable posterior horn tears approaching the midline.

All-inside repair is particularly useful for repairable posterior horn tears approaching the midline (Fig. **2a-b**). No open posterior capsular exposure is required. Improved devices are versatile and allow for mattress suture configuration most zones. Biomechanically equivalent outcomes to standard vertical mattress repairs have been reported with later-generation devices. However, the stability of these repair devices requires an intact meniscocapsular junction, therefore a frank meniscocapsular separation is a contraindication to their use. Moreover, access for anterior zone repairs is extremely difficult and is better suited for repair with outside-in techniques [49]. The post-operative care is obviously conditioned by the fracture post-operative protocol. There is no total agreement on the rehabilitation protocol for meniscus repairs, but in most of the conventional rehabilitation protocols weightbearing is not allowed for the first 3-4 weeks, and usually a 4-week period of restricted ROM (until 90°) is recommended [50]. However, this kind of rehabilitation protocol is overwhelmed by the post-operative protocol for tibial plateau fracture, with usually a minimum of 8 weeks without weight bearing.

Ligamentous Tears: Timing, Treatment and Post-Operative Care

As previously stated, the correct treatment of ligamentous tears associated to tibial plateau fractures is still debated and not completely clear. Agreement is widespread that ligamentous injuries associated with bony avulsion should be acutely repaired at the time of operative fracture fixation [51].

Delamarter *et al.* reported the poor prognosis of concomitant ACL injury and tibial plateau fracture. They found a high incidence of ACL residual laxity and recommended reduction and fixation of involved intercondylar eminences at the time of plateau fixation [52] (Fig. **3a-b**). In the absence of bony avulsion, ligament augmentation and reconstruction often are complicated by the presence of the fracture and the fixation methods, therefore functional and residual laxity should be addressed at a later date.

Egol *et al.* recommended treating midsubstance ACL tears at a later date if residual laxity remains [53]. Regarding midsubstance MCL tears, Egol *et al.* recommended "conservative, nonoperative treatment because the surgical exposure and postoperative immobilization required can lead to stiffness" and other undesirable outcomes [53]. Moreover, is well established that isolated tears of MCL, even when they are complete tears, can heal with nonoperative treatment reaching an excellent outcome [54]. "However, it is well established that many ligament injuries have better functional outcomes with surgical treatments, such as ACL tears in active patients, multiligament knee injuries, and PLC tears" [26].

"Although the treatment of collateral ligament tears remains controversial, it is generally agreed that anterior cruciate ligament (ACL) avulsions need to be repaired acutely in order to maintain knee joint stability, while reconstruction of cruciate ligament tears is typically deferred after osseous healing" [25, 38].

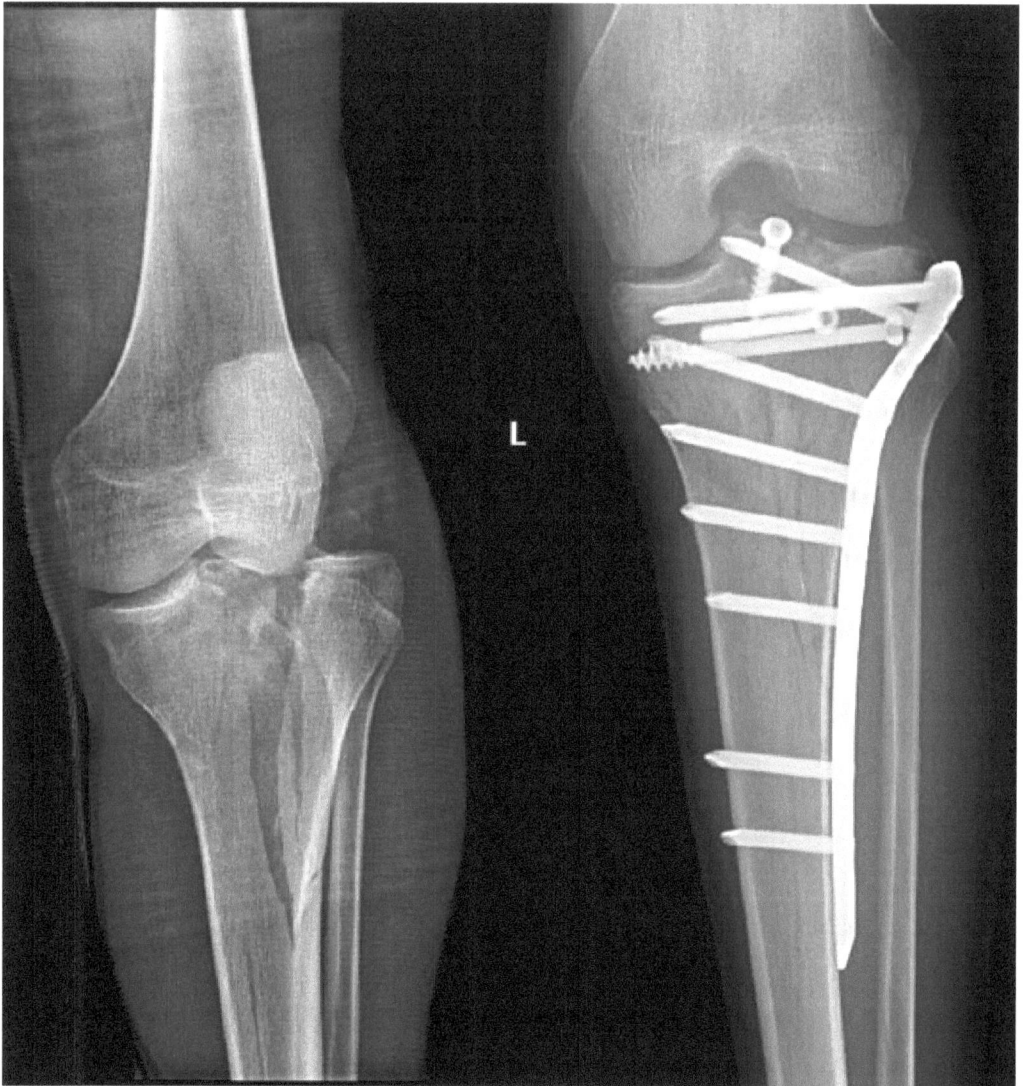

Fig. (3). Reduction and fixation of involved intercondylar eminences at the time of plateau fixation is recommended.

Lesions of the posterior cruciate ligament are much less frequent (0%–15%). They are generally treated conservatively or, if necessary, by delayed secondary reconstruction [42].

In a retrospective study performed on 29 MRI scans of 29 patients with acute tibial plateau fractures, Colletti *et al.* reported that 12 (41%) patients had complete

(8) or partial (4) anterior cruciate ligament injuries while only 8 (28%) patients had complete (3) or partial (5) posterior cruciate ligament injuries. Sprained (10) or torn (6) medial collateral ligaments were noted in 16 (55%) patients. The lateral collateral ligament was sprained (3) or torn (7) in 10 (34%) patients.

The three most common injuries associated with lateral plateau fractures were MCL injuries (55%), lateral meniscus tears (45%) and ACL (41%) injuries. Avulsion of the attachment of the ACL occurred in 27% of the ACL disruptions [28].

In a prospective cohort study on 103 patients with operative tibial plateau fractures, Gardner *et al.* reported that 79 patients (77%) sustained a complete tear or avulsion of 1 or more cruciate or collateral ligaments, and 70 patients (68%) had tears of 1 or more of the posterolateral corner structures of the knee [31].

In a series of 54 patients who received arthroscopy-assisted surgery for tibial plateau fractures, Chan *et al.* reported that 35 of them (65%) had associated intra-articular lesions. Ligament injuries were noted in 22 knees with 24 lesions including 11 ACL avulsion fractures, 3 ACL partial ruptures, 5 posterior cruciate ligament partial ruptures, 2 medial collateral ligament partial ruptures, and 3 lateral collateral ligament (LCL) avulsions in the fibular insertion. There were 2 combined ligament injuries (ACL and medial collateral ligament partial rupture in 1 and ACL and LCL avulsion fracture in 1). 11 ACL avulsions were treated by arthroscopic suture fixation. The LCL avulsion was fixed with a screw and washer [7].

In 98 cases of tibial plateau fractures which underwent to arthroscopic evaluation of soft tissue injuries, Abdel-Hamid *et al.* reported that "the second most common soft tissue injury was ACL injury in 25% of the fractures and consisted of 10 tibial avulsion treated by arthroscopically assisted fixation by cancellous screws or pullout suture, 10 cases of partial tear, treated by arthroscopic shaving and debridement, and 4 cases of midsubstance rupture, treated by second-stage reconstruction following fracture healing. The sample included 5 (5%) posterior cruciate ligament (PCL) injuries (2 avulsion fractures, treated by arthroscopically assisted fixation by pullout suture, 2 midsubstance ruptures, treated by second-stage reconstruction following fracture healing, and 1 partial tear, treated by arthroscopic shaving and debridement). The study sample included 3 cases (3%) of MCL injury (2 cases of partial tear, treated conservatively, and 1 case of avulsion fracture of the femoral site insertion, treated by screw fixation), 3 cases (3%) of LCL injury (1 case of partial tear, treated nonoperatively, 1 case of avulsion fracture of the femoral site insertion, treated by screw fixation, and 1 case of complete tear, treated by suture fixation)" [1].

Stannard *et al.* reported that in their group "71% of 103 tibial plateau fractures after high-energy trauma had at least one ligament injury (diagnosed on MRI scans), while 53% of these patients had multiple ligament injuries. 27 patients had knee dislocations with complete ACL and PCL tear, without showing on initial radiographs a dislocated joint. 45 patients reported an ACL tear, 41 a PCL tear, 46 a PLC (postero-lateral corner) injury, 16 a PMC (postero-medial corner) injury.

Both Schatzker V and VI fractures had a higher incidence of ligament tears than that of Schatzker IV fractures. However, the medial tibial plateau fractures had the highest incidence of PCL tears (54%), PLC tears (62%), and bicruciate injuries or knee dislocations (46%)" [26].

In their systematic review, including 19 articles with 609 patients (610 knees) with tibial plateau fractures, Chen *et al.* reported that 119 patients (21.3%) had ACL injuries, and that ACL midsubstance injuries were not operated on in the same procedure, but ACL bony avulsions were treated with arthroscopy-assisted fixation during the same operation [2] .

In conclusion, only ligamentous injuries associated to bony avulsion must be acutely repaired at the time of operative fracture fixation. The fixation can be performed with trans-osseous suture fixation or by (usually cannulated and half-threaded) screw fixation. When treating cruciate ligaments bony avulsions (intercondylar eminence avulsion fractures), disadvantages of screw fixation include risks of comminution of the fracture fragment, posterior neurovascular injury, and the need for hardware removal. Because of these risks, ARIF using nonabsorbable sutures passed through drill holes and tied over the tibial tubercle is often preferred [55] (Fig. **4a-b**). For collateral ligaments bony avulsions, screw fixation (Fig. **5a-b**) with a cannulated screw and a washer (with or without spikes) is usually more likely.

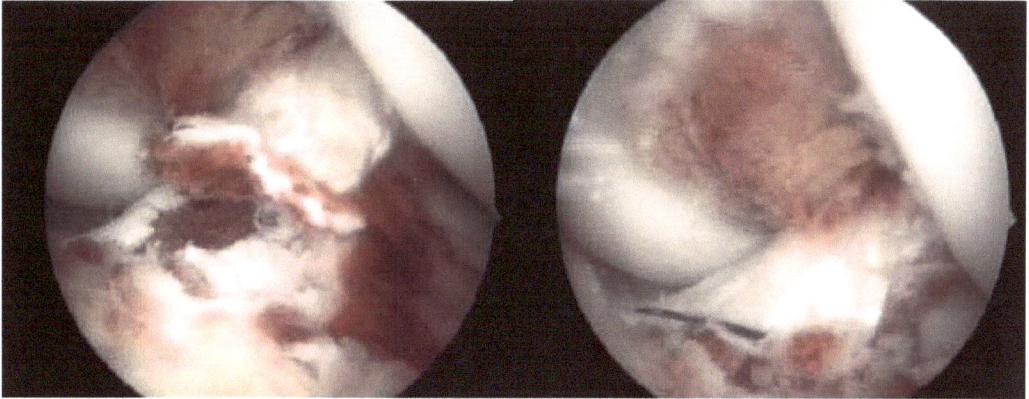

Fig. (4). When treating cruciate ligaments bony avulsions, ARIF using nonabsorbable sutures passed through drill holes and tied over the tibial tubercle is often preferred.

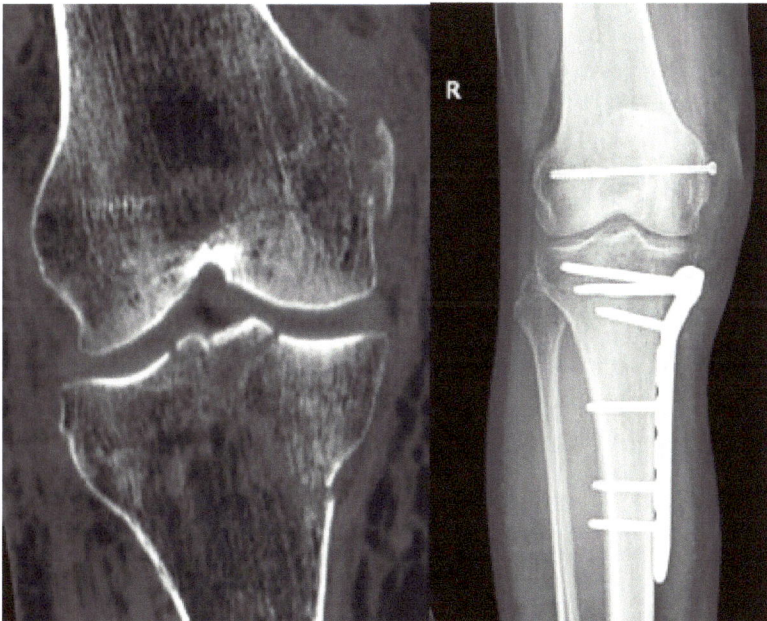

Fig. (5). Schatzker type IV tibial plateau fracture with MCL bony avulsion at the femoral side:fixation with a half-threaded cannulated screw.

Post-operative care must achieve the goal of full range of motion of the knee by six weeks. Usually the post-operative protocol does not interfere with the fracture healing, full weightbearing not being allowed before 12 weeks after surgery. Early active and passive motion of the knee is recommended, especially in case of ligamentous repair associated to tibial plateau fracture fixation, to avoid stiffness [26].

COPYRIGHT LETTER

The chapter is prepared according to the *'Guidelines for Authors'*. The chapter does not contain any such material or information that may be unlawful, defamatory, fabricated, plagiarized, or which would, if published, in any way whatsoever, violate the terms and conditions as laid down in the Copyright letter.

CONFLICT OF INTEREST

The author confirms that author has no conflict of interest to declare for this publication.

ACKNOWLEDGEMENTS

Declared none.

REFERENCES

[1]   Abdel-Hamid MZ, Chang CH, Chan YS, *et al.* Arthroscopic evaluation of soft tissue injuries in tibial plateau fractures: retrospective analysis of 98 cases. Arthroscopy 2006; 22(6): 669-75.
[http://dx.doi.org/10.1016/j.arthro.2006.01.018] [PMID: 16762707]

[2]   Chen XZ, Liu CG, Chen Y, Wang LQ, Zhu QZ, Lin P. Arthroscopy-Assisted Surgery for Tibial Plateau Fractures 2014.

[3]   Burdin G. Arthroscopic management of tibial plateau fractures: surgical technique. Orthop Traumatol Surg Res 2013; 99(1) (Suppl.): S208-18.
[http://dx.doi.org/10.1016/j.otsr.2012.11.011] [PMID: 23347755]

[4]   Cetik O, Cift H, Asik M. Second-look arthroscopy after arthroscopy-assisted treatment of tibial plateau fractures. Knee Surg Sports Traumatol Arthrosc 2007; 15(6): 747-52.
[http://dx.doi.org/10.1007/s00167-006-0276-6] [PMID: 17225173]

[5]   Rademakers MV, Kerkhoffs GM, Sierevelt IN, Raaymakers EL, Marti RK. Operative treatment of 109 tibial plateau fractures: five- to 27-year follow-up results. J Orthop Trauma 2007; 21(1): 5-10.
[http://dx.doi.org/10.1097/BOT.0b013e31802c5b51] [PMID: 17211262]

[6]   Lubowitz JH, Elson WS, Guttmann D, Part I. Part I: Arthroscopic management of tibial plateau fractures. Arthroscopy 2004; 20(10): 1063-70.
[http://dx.doi.org/10.1016/j.arthro.2004.09.001] [PMID: 15592236]

[7]   Chan YS, Chiu CH, Lo YP, *et al.* Arthroscopy-assisted surgery for tibial plateau fractures: 2- to 10-year follow-up results. Arthroscopy 2008; 24(7): 760-8.
[http://dx.doi.org/10.1016/j.arthro.2008.02.017] [PMID: 18589264]

[8]   Kennedy JC, Bailey WH. Experimental tibial-plateau fractures. Studies of the mechanism and a classification. J Bone Joint Surg Am 1968; 50(8): 1522-34.
[PMID: 5722848]

[9]   Foltin E. Bone loss and forms of tibial condylar fracture. Arch Orthop Trauma Surg 1987; 106(6): 341-8.
[http://dx.doi.org/10.1007/BF00456867] [PMID: 3435233]

[10]   Foltin E. Osteoporosis and fracture patterns. A study of split-compression fractures of the lateral tibial condyle. Int Orthop 1988; 12(4): 299-303.
[http://dx.doi.org/10.1007/BF00317828] [PMID: 3220622]

[11]   Borrelli J Jr. Management of soft tissue injuries associated with tibial plateau fractures. J Knee Surg 2014; 27(1): 5-9.
[PMID: 24357043]

[12]   Kobbe P, Pape HC.

[13]   Schaser KD, Vollmar B, Menger MD, *et al. In vivo* analysis of microcirculation following closed soft-tissue injury. J Orthop Res 1999; 17(5): 678-85.
[http://dx.doi.org/10.1002/jor.1100170509] [PMID: 10569476]

[14]   Sudkamp NP. Soft-tissue injury: pathophysiology and its influence on fracture management. In: Reudi TP, Murphy WM, Eds. AO principles of fracture management. Stuttgart, Germany: Thieme Verlag 2000; pp. 59-77.

[15]   Gardner AM, Fox RH. The venous footpump: influence on tissue perfusion and prevention of venous thrombosis. Ann Rheum Dis 1992; 51(10): 1173-8.
[http://dx.doi.org/10.1136/ard.51.10.1173] [PMID: 1444634]

[16]   Gardner AM, Fox RH, Lawrence C, Bunker TD, Ling RS, MacEachern AG. Reduction of post-traumatic swelling and compartment pressure by impulse compression of the foot. J Bone Joint Surg Br 1990; 72(5): 810-5.
[PMID: 2211762]

[17]   McMaster WC, Liddle S. Cryotherapy influence on posttraumatic limb edema. Clin Orthop Relat Res 1980; 150(150): 283-7.
[PMID: 7428234]

[18]   Webb JM, Williams D, Ivory JP, Day S, Williamson DM. The use of cold compression dressings after total knee replacement: a randomized controlled trial. Orthopedics 1998; 21(1): 59-61.
[PMID: 9474633]

[19]   Healy WL, Seidman J, Pfeifer BA, Brown DG. Cold compressive dressing after total knee arthroplasty. Clin Orthop Relat Res 1994; 299(299): 143-6.
[PMID: 7907012]

[20]   Barei DP, Nork SE, Mills WJ, Henley MB, Benirschke SK. Complications associated with internal fixation of high-energy bicondylar tibial plateau fractures utilizing a two-incision technique. J Orthop

Trauma 2004; 18(10): 649-57.
[http://dx.doi.org/10.1097/00005131-200411000-00001] [PMID: 15507817]

[21] Barei DP, Nork SE, Mills WJ, Coles CP, Henley MB, Benirschke SK. Functional outcomes of severe bicondylar tibial plateau fractures treated with dual incisions and medial and lateral plates. J Bone Joint Surg Am 2006; 88(8): 1713-21.
[http://dx.doi.org/10.2106/JBJS.E.00907] [PMID: 16882892]

[22] Risko TM, Ricci WM.

[23] Inaba K, Potzman J, Munera F, *et al.* Multi-slice CT angiography for arterial evaluation in the injured lower extremity. J Trauma 2006; 60(3): 502-6.
[http://dx.doi.org/10.1097/01.ta.0000204150.78156.a9] [PMID: 16531846]

[24] Holt MD, Williams LA, Dent CM. MRI in the management of tibial plateau fractures. Injury 1995; 26(9): 595-9.
[http://dx.doi.org/10.1016/0020-1383(95)00109-M] [PMID: 8550164]

[25] Gardner MJ, Yacoubian S, Geller D, *et al.* The incidence of soft tissue injury in operative tibial plateau fractures: a magnetic resonance imaging analysis of 103 patients. J Orthop Trauma 2005; 19(2): 79-84.
[http://dx.doi.org/10.1097/00005131-200502000-00002] [PMID: 15677922]

[26] Stannard JP, Lopez R, Volgas D. Soft tissue injury of the knee after tibial plateau fractures. J Knee Surg 2010; 23(4): 187-92.
[http://dx.doi.org/10.1055/s-0030-1268694] [PMID: 21446623]

[27] Ip D. 2008.

[28] Colletti P, Greenberg H, Terk MR. MR findings in patients with acute tibial plateau fractures. Comput Med Imaging Graph 1996; 20(5): 389-94.
[http://dx.doi.org/10.1016/S0895-6111(96)00054-7] [PMID: 9007366]

[29] Shepherd L, Abdollahi K, Lee J, Vangsness CT Jr. The prevalence of soft tissue injuries in nonoperative tibial plateau fractures as determined by magnetic resonance imaging. J Orthop Trauma 2002; 16(9): 628-31.
[http://dx.doi.org/10.1097/00005131-200210000-00003] [PMID: 12368642]

[30] Asik M, Cetik O, Talu U, Sozen YV. Arthroscopy-assisted operative management of tibial plateau fractures. Knee Surg Sports Traumatol Arthrosc 2002; 10(6): 364-70.
[http://dx.doi.org/10.1007/s00167-002-0310-2] [PMID: 12444516]

[31] Gardner MJ, Yacoubian S, Geller D, *et al.* The incidence of soft tissue injury in operative tibial plateau fractures: a magnetic resonance imaging analysis of 103 patients. J Orthop Trauma 2005; 19(2): 79-84.
[http://dx.doi.org/10.1097/00005131-200502000-00002] [PMID: 15677922]

[32] Mustonen AO, Koivikko MP, Lindahl J, Koskinen SK. MRI of acute meniscal injury associated with tibial plateau fractures: prevalence, type, and location. AJR Am J Roentgenol 2008; 191(4): 1002-9.
[http://dx.doi.org/10.2214/AJR.07.3811] [PMID: 18806134]

[33] Urruela AM, Davidovitch R, Karia R, Khurana S, Egol KA. Results following operative treatment of tibial plateau fractures. J Knee Surg 2013; 26(3): 161-5.
[http://dx.doi.org/10.1055/s-0032-1324807] [PMID: 23288754]

[34] Spiro AS, Regier M, Novo de Oliveira A, *et al.* The degree of articular depression as a predictor of soft-tissue injuries in tibial plateau fracture. Knee Surg Sports Traumatol Arthrosc 2013; 21(3): 564-70.
[http://dx.doi.org/10.1007/s00167-012-2201-5] [PMID: 22965381]

[35] Wiss DA, Watson JT. Fractures of the tibial plateau. In: Rockwood CA, Green DP, Bucholz RW, Heckman JD, Eds. Rockwood and Green's fractures in adults. Philadelphia: Lippincott-Raven 1996; pp. 1920-53.

[36] Lobenhoffer P, Schulze M, Gerich T, Lattermann C, Tscherne H. Closed reduction/percutaneous fixation of tibial plateau fractures: arthroscopic *versus* fluoroscopic control of reduction. J Orthop Trauma 1999; 13(6): 426-31.
[http://dx.doi.org/10.1097/00005131-199908000-00006] [PMID: 10459602]

[37] Fischbach R, Prokop A, Maintz D, Zähringer M, Landwehr P. Magnetic resonance tomography in the diagnosis of intra-articular tibial plateau fractures: value of fracture classification and spectrum of fracture associated soft tissue injuries. Rofo 2000; 172(7): 597-603. Magnetic resonance tomography in the diagnosis of intra-articular tibial plateau fractures: value of fracture classification and spectrum of fracture associated soft tissue injuries. [Article in German].
[http://dx.doi.org/10.1055/s-2000-4649] [PMID: 10962985]

[38] Mui LW, Engelsohn E, Umans H. Comparison of CT and MRI in patients with tibial plateau fracture: can CT findings predict ligament tear or meniscal injury? Skeletal Radiol 2007; 36(2): 145-51.
[http://dx.doi.org/10.1007/s00256-006-0216-z] [PMID: 17136560]

[39] Gardner MJ, Yacoubian S, Geller D, *et al.* Prediction of soft-tissue injuries in Schatzker II tibial plateau fractures based on measurements of plain radiographs. J Trauma 2006; 60(2): 319-23.
[http://dx.doi.org/10.1097/01.ta.0000203548.50829.92] [PMID: 16508489]

[40] Ringus VM, Lemley FR, Hubbard DF, Wearden S, Jones DL. Lateral tibial plateau fracture depression as a predictor of lateral meniscus pathology. Orthopedics 2010; 33(2): 80-4.
[http://dx.doi.org/10.3928/01477447-20100104-05] [PMID: 20192139]

[41] Durakbasa MO, Kose O, Ermis MN, Demirtas A, Gunday S, Islam C. Measurement of lateral plateau depression and lateral plateau widening in a Schatzker type II fracture can predict a lateral meniscal injury. Knee Surg Sports Traumatol Arthrosc 2013; 21(9): 2141-6.
[http://dx.doi.org/10.1007/s00167-012-2195-z] [PMID: 22956166]

[42] Handelberg FWJ, Scheerlinck T, Casteleyn PP. Fractures of the Upper Tibia and Arthroscopic Techniques. Techniques in Knee Surgery 2003; 2(2): 109-16.
[http://dx.doi.org/10.1097/00132588-200306000-00006]

[43] Tejwani NC. Arthroscopic assisted management of tibial plateau fractures. Tech Knee Surg 2005; 4(4): 237-41.
[http://dx.doi.org/10.1097/01.btk.0000187523.78209.dd]

[44] Honkonen SE. Degenerative arthritis after tibial plateau fractures. J Orthop Trauma 1995; 9(4): 273-7.
[http://dx.doi.org/10.1097/00005131-199509040-00001] [PMID: 7562147]

[45] Chan YS, Yuan LJ, Hung SS, *et al.* Arthroscopic-assisted reduction with bilateral buttress plate fixation of complex tibial plateau fractures. Arthroscopy 2003; 19(9): 974-84.

[http://dx.doi.org/10.1016/j.arthro.2003.09.038] [PMID: 14608317]

[46] Ruiz-Ibán MÁ, Diaz-Heredia J, Elías-Martín E, Moros-Marco S, Cebreiro Martinez Del Val I. Repair of meniscal tears associated with tibial plateau fractures: a review of 15 cases. Am J Sports Med 2012; 40(10): 2289-95.
[http://dx.doi.org/10.1177/0363546512457552] [PMID: 22962298]

[47] Forman JM, Karia RJ, Davidovitch RI, Egol KA. Tibial plateau fractures with and without meniscus tear-results of a standardized treatment protocol. Bull Hosp Jt Dis 2013; 71(2): 144-51.

[48] Jouve F, Ovadia H, Pujol N, Beaufils P. Chapter 43: Meniscal Repair: Technique. Verlag Berlin Heidelberg: The Meniscus Springer 2010.

[49] Bedi A, Warren RF. Techniques of Meniscal Repair. Gill TJ, Andrews JR, David TS: Arthroscopic Techniques of the Knee – A visual guide. Slack Incorporated 2009.

[50] Witvrouw E, Thijs Y. Chapter 46: Rehabilitation. Verlag Berlin Heidelberg: The Meniscus Springer 2010.

[51] Ziran BH, Hooks B, Pesantez R. Complex fractures of the tibial plateau. J Knee Surg 2007; 20(1): 67-77.
[PMID: 17288092]

[52] Delamarter RB, Hohl M, Hopp E Jr. Ligament injuries associated with tibial plateau fractures. Clin Orthop Relat Res 1990; (250): 226-33.
[PMID: 2293934]

[53] Egol KA, Tejwani NC, Capla EL, Wolinsky PL, Koval KJ. Staged management of high-energy proximal tibia fractures (OTA types 41): the results of a prospective, standardized protocol. J Orthop Trauma 2005; 19(7): 448-55.
[http://dx.doi.org/10.1097/01.bot.0000171881.11205.80] [PMID: 16056075]

[54] Indelicato PA. Non-operative treatment of complete tears of the medial collateral ligament of the knee. J Bone Joint Surg Am 1983; 65(3): 323-9.
[PMID: 6826594]

[55] Lubowitz JH, Elson WS, Guttmann D, Part II. Part II: arthroscopic treatment of tibial plateau fractures: intercondylar eminence avulsion fractures. Arthroscopy 2005; 21(1): 86-92.
[http://dx.doi.org/10.1016/j.arthro.2004.09.031] [PMID: 15650672]

CHAPTER 10

The Role of Primary Total Knee Arthroplasty (TKA) in Tibial Plateau Fractures

Federica Rosso[1], Umberto Cottino[1], Matteo Bruzzone[2], Federico Dettoni[2], Davide Deledda[1] and **Roberto Rossi[2,*]**

[1] *School of Orthopaedics and Traumatology, University of Turin, (Turin), Italy*

[2] *University of Turin, Department of Orthopaedic and Traumatology, Hospital Mauriziano Umberto I, Largo Turati 62, 10128 Torino (TO), Italy*

Abstract: Total Knee Arthroplasties (TKAs) in tibial plateau fractures can be performed in the acute or chronic settings. Treatment of tibial plateau fractures with Open reduction and Internal Fixation (ORIF) in elderly patients can lead to poor results because of poor bone quality, fracture complexity and higher risk of complications. For these reasons primary TKA in the acute setting can be an option in elderly patients. Most of the authors agree in confirming that this is a safe treatment with good clinical outcomes, but inferior compared to whom obtained in elective TKAs, with a higher risk of complications, similar to those reported in revision TKAs. On the other hand ORIF is the gold standard treatment in tibial plateau fractures in younger patients, but the incidence of post-traumatic arthritis is high, with the need of TKA conversion. There are few reports on literature on TKAs performed after tibial plateau fractures, but there is agreement in affirming that clinical outcomes and implant survival in those cases are lower than in TKA performed for primary arthritis. In this chapter we will analyze the indication for primary TKR in tibial plateau fractures, both in acute and chronic setting, with a literature review on the clinical outcomes.

Keywords: Arthritis, Arthroplasty, Elderly, Fracture, Knee, Post-traumatic, Tibial plateau.

* **Correspondence author Roberto Rossi:** Department of Orthopedic and Traumatology, Largo Turati 62, 10128, Torino Italy; Tel +390115082317; E-mail: rrossi@fastwebnet.it

Francesco Atzori and Luigi Sabatini (Eds)

INTRODUCTION

The tibial plateau fractures represent 1-2% of all fractures, with an annual incidence of 13.3 per 100000 in the adult population; however approximately 50% of those fractures occur in patient older than 50 years old, with 8% to 24% occurring in elderly. In the elderly those fractures can result from a low energy trauma, with greater prevalence in man (male female ratio 54:46) [1]. The goals of treatment in these cases are: 1) pain control, 2) early mobilization, 3) restoration of function and 4) minimizing the need for further surgery. In young patients Open Reduction and Internal Fixation (ORIF) is the gold standard [2]. In some cases primary Total Knee Arthroplasty (TKA) may play a role in tibial plateau fractures treatment. In this chapter we will analyze the role of TKA both in the acute and chronic setting, in association to indication, surgical technique and results.

ACUTE SETTING

Introduction

ORIF is often the treatment of choice in tibial plateau fractures [2]. However there is still a concern in using ORIF in elderly patients, because of poor bone quality, fracture complexity and higher risk of complications [3]. Honkonen underlined the difficulties to obtain a stable fixation in elderly patients, in association to the high risk of losing reduction despite stable internal fixation and bone grafting [4]. Although poor fixation may be improved with newer angle-stable plate, adequate reduction remains challenging. Besides soft tissue stripping needed for ORIF may lead to wound healing problems. Finally most type of fracture fixation do not allow immediate post-operative weight-bearing [5]. For those reasons some authors described an unacceptable failure rate (79%) and unsatisfactory results for ORIF in elderly patients [6].

The main complications reported on literature for ORIF are loss of fixation, post-traumatic arthritis requiring TKA, malunion or nonunion, stiffness and medical co-morbidities secondary to immobilization. Besides TKA in patients with previous tibial plateau fractures is challenging because of the difficulty ligament balancing, extensor mechanism scars, patellar maltracking and the need to restore a better lower limb alignment. 26% of complications have been reported for TKAs in patients with a previous tibial plateau fracture, with a reoperation rate of 21% [7]. Those complications, associated to the need of early mobilization, have led several authors to recently suggest the use of TKA for acute treatment of tibial plateau fracture in elderly [3, 8 - 13]. Primary TKA in tibial plateau fractures seems to have better functional outcomes, better survival and lower complications rate if compared to ORIF in the elderly, also if the results cannot not achieve those obtained with TKA in primary osteoarthritis [3].

Indication

Primary cemented TKA may be an option in acute treatment of elderly patient affected by proximal tibial fractures due to previous osteoarthritis, with the main advantage of early mobilization compared to ORIF. However, mechanical failure, loosening and periprosthetic fractures are still a concern; for these reasons it should be reserved to elderly sedentary patients [14]. Surgeons should take in consideration managing acute tibial plateau fracture with TKA in patients with pre-existing arthritis, who are unable to comply with restricted weight-bearing, with comminuted type C intra-articular fractures and in patients in whom a secondary procedure is best avoided [8]. A relative contraindication to primary TKA in tibial plateau fracture is avulsion of the tibial tubercle, because nonunion of this fragment after TKA is really demanding to manage [3, 15].

Pre-Operative Planning

In acute trauma the pre-operative planning is more difficult compared to elective TKA, because there are no weight-bearing X-rays, so the radiological alignment is difficult to evaluated. Antero-posterior and lateral x-ray on rest are mandatory; Computer Tomography (CT) scan is really useful to classify the fracture morphology and to identify the amount of bone losses [16]. Clinical evaluation of medial-lateral instability is fundamental to help the surgeon in deciding the grade of constrain, that should be planned pre-operatively [8].

Surgical Technique

There are few differences in elective or acute trauma TKA in terms of surgical technique.

First the surgeon should plan the incision in order to enable the addition of any internal fixation; a midline incision is often the best choice [3, 8, 16]. Joint line restoration and assessment of component rotation can be more challenging compared to elective primary TKA, particularly in patients with major epiphyseal bone deficiency. Temporary fracture reduction can help in identifying correct joint line and components rotation using standard anatomical landmarks (medial epicondyle, trans-epicondylar line *etc.*). If it cannot be obtained, surgeons can apply the rules used in revision TKAs, for example using the lower pole of the patella [11, 17]. Once the joint line has been assessed, bone cutting is performed taking care to preserve as much bone as possible. Some authors suggested using an intramedullary alignment both on the femoral and tibial cuts to simplify conversion to stemmed implants if necessary [3, 8].

To size the femoral and tibial component the same rules used in revision TKA can be applied: bone losses should not be considered and the contra-lateral knee can be used to identify the correct size and to avoid too large extension or flexion gaps [17].

The other points that must be considered approaching to a primary TKA in proximal tibial fractures are the grade of constrain, the use of stem and how to manage bony defect.

The minimum amount of constrained should be used in order to achieve stability of the knee minimizing the risk of loosening, as well as in revision TKA [3, 8].

Different authors suggested using uncemented intramedullary stems, overall on the tibial side, in order to obtain a better fixation in cases with associated bone defects. Besides some authors suggested using longer stem in case of diaphyseal fractures, like an intramedullary fixation [12]. However there is some agreement in using tibial stem in case of C-types fractures involving the metaphyseal region and in case of higher constrained implants, while some split-depression fractures can be treated with standard implants [10]. Some authors suggested avoiding femoral stem if possible, overall in patients with ipsilateral hip arthroplasty, because the limit between the proximal and distal femoral stem is a weak point, and there is an increase in peri-prosthetic fracture risk [10].

There are different options for tibial bone defects managing in these cases, including cement, cement with screw augmentation, metallic wedges, bone autograft or allograft, sleeves, cone-shape augments and custom-made prostheses. However, most of the authors agree to treat contained defect less than 5 mm with cement, and greater defect using metallic augments, bone graft or tantalium cones in case of metaphyseal defect [12].

Bohm *et al.* suggested that fracture fragments must be stably fixed and protected with intramedullary stems, in order to allow early weight-bearing. Besides they suggested an algorithm based on Schatzker classification. In Schatzker type III fractures, with depression of the lateral tibial plateau, the defects smaller than 1 cm can be filled with cement, or using a cancellous bone graft if it is larger. In these cases, in there is good circumferential cortical bone stock, superficial prosthesis without stems can be used. In presence of uncontained bone defects, tibial augments and stems are mandatory to restore the metaphyseal support and to guarantee a stable fixation.

For unicondylar fractures (Schatzker types I, II, IV), the authors suggested using intramedullary fixation, supplemented by internal fixation if the fragments are large enough. Finally Schatzker type V and VI that involve both condyles, with or without metaphyseal extension, are the most demanding fractures to manage, and the authors suggested a combination of tibial stems and plate fixation [3].

Patellar replacement is still debated, but some authors suggested to be reasonable to replace it in these cases to reduce the risk of needed for further surgery [3].

(Fig. **1**) shows the case of a 80 years-old female affected by complex tibial plateau fracture and treated with primary TKA in the acute setting. In this case the surgeon temporarily fixed the fractures with some Kirshner wires and then implanted a constrained prosthesis (RHK Zimmer®, Warsaw).

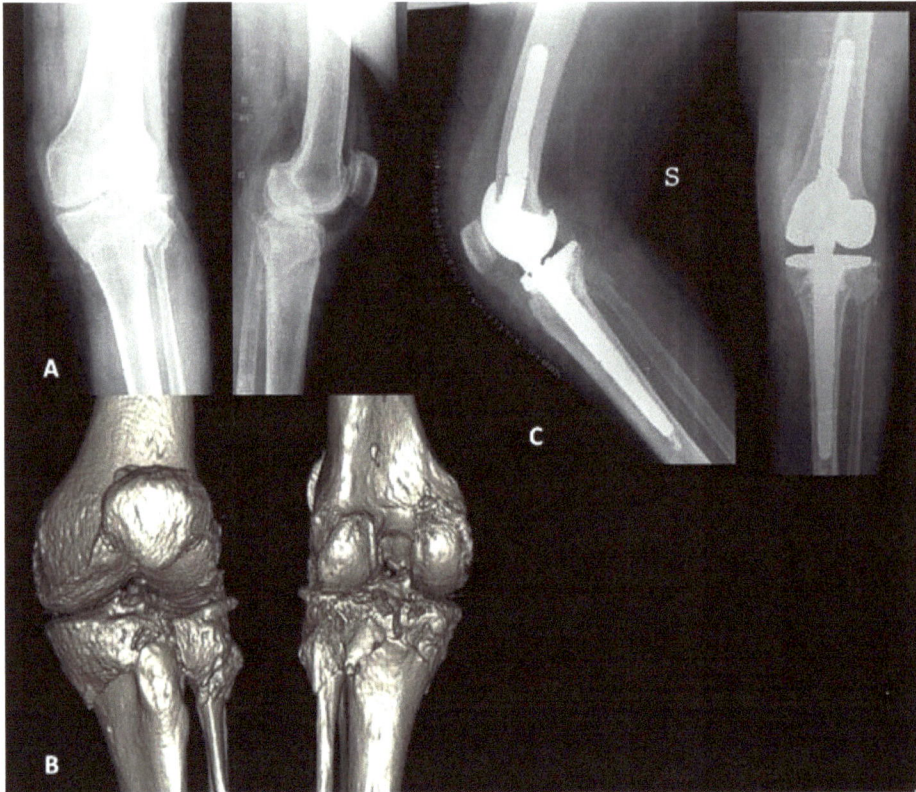

Fig. (1). A) X-ray evalutaion of a 80 years old female with proximal tibial plateau fracture. B) 3D CT scan of the same case. C) post-operative x-rays showing the constrained TKA correctly implanted).

Results

There are few reports on literature describing the outcomes of primary TKA in tibial plateau fractures. However there is some agreement in affirming that, although primary hip arthroplasty for proximal femoral fractures is a well-accepted treatment, this is not the case of TKA [10].

The first report on literature of TKAs performed acutely in proximal tibial fractures is the one from Nau *et al.* in 2003, describing their results on 6 patients, with 5 of them receiving a rotating-hinge implant. They concluded describing moderate functional outcomes, with the knee flexion ranging from 70° to 110° and only 2 patients pain free [13].

Nourissat *et al.* in 2004 described their results in 4 patients, with three excellent

IKS outcomes, concluding that primary arthroplasty for complex tibial plateau fractures is a realistic option [18].

Vermiere *et al.* described the bigger casuistry in literature, with 12 patients affected by complex proximal tibial fractures treated with primary TKA, with good functional outcomes. The authors concluded that primary TKA in complex proximal tibial fractures with or without a metaphyseal component is a safe procedure resulting in acceptable results, but it should be reserved to elderly patients or in those affected by pre-existing osteoarthritis [10].

Parratte *et al.* described the results in 26 patients treated in different centers in France, including 10 patients affected by distal femoral fractures and 16 patients by proximal tibial one. They reported 23% of immediate general and 15% of locale knee-related complications, and concluded that primary TKA is a suitable option for complex proximal tibial fracture in elderly patients suffering of osteoarthritis, with higher complication rate compared to elective TKA but comparable to those observed after post-traumatic arthritis [11].

Malviya *et al.* reported on their results in acute TKA for peri-articular knee fractures in patients over 65 years of age (both distal femoral and proximal tibial fractures). The authors concluded that primary TKAs in proximal tibial fractures should be considered as a treatment option in elderly with osteoporosis and/or osteoarthritis [9].

Kini *et al.* in 2013 described their results in 9 knees (6 affected by a lateral tibial plateau fractures and 3 by diaphyseal fractures) treated with primary navigated TKAs. In 5 on 6 patients with proximal tibial fractures a postero-stabilized implant was used, while in the cases affected by diaphyseal fractures longer tibial stems were used. In this casuistry the average Knee Society Score was 84, with 5 patients out of 9 graded as excellent [12].

Finally Benazzo *et al.* in 2014 reported their results on 6 knees affected both by distal femoral or proximal tibial fractures and treated acutely with TKAs. They described good outcomes in both groups with an average follow-up of 12 months [8]. Table **1** shows in summary these results.

Table 1. Literature review describing in detail the results in patients affected by proximal tibial plateau fractures and treated with primary Total Knee Arthroplasty (TKA).

Authors	Year	Number of knees	Average age	Type of implants	Mean follow-up	Results
Nau *et al.* (13)	2003	6 knees	79 years (range 70-90)	5 patients: Link Endo-Model Rotation Knee Joint Prosthesis (Link®). 1 patient: unconstrained Alpina CR (Biomet®)	24.4 months	No loosening at follow-up evaluation. 4 patients reported mild or occasional pain at follow-up evaluation. All patients had full extension. In 5 cases, the knee flexion ranged from 70°to 110°. Four women needed a cane, and the remaining 2 needed walkers.
Nourissat *et al.* (18)	2006	4 knees	Over 75 years old	Constrained implants in all cases, long-stem, cemented tibial componenent when epiphysis reconstruction.	2 to 7 years	Excellent IKS for three knees (90, 95, 95). All x-rays showed bone healing with aligned limbs (less than 2 degrees deformation). There were no lucent lines at last follow-up.
Schwarz *et al.* (37)	2008	10 knees	55-85 years	One unilateral, three superficial, and six revision-type prostheses.	6 months to 3 years	One deep infection treated with arthroscopic lavage. At last follow-up all eight patients were completely or almost pain free; the extension deficit was less than 10 degrees, and flexion was 100 degrees or more.
Vermeire *et al.* (10)	2010	12 knees	73 years (range 53-81)	11/12 cemented posterior stabilized and 1/12 constrained condylar TKA with a stemmed tibial component bypassing the fracture area. The stem was cemented in 2 cases, graft impaction in 5 and augmentation block in 2. In 7 cases additional fixation of the tibial plateau was performed.	31 months	9 patients with normal alignment and 2 with valgus one. The mean knee flexion was 115.9° (95-130°). 5 patients were free from pain. The median final knee score was 78 points(range : 50-100) and the median function score 58 (range : 0-100). 7 patients were rated as excellent. Radiologically, no signs of loosening were seen and no implant revisions were necessary

(Table 1) contd.....

Authors	Year	Number of knees	Average age	Type of implants	Mean follow-up	Results
Parratte *et al.* (11)	2011	26 knees (16 proximal tibial fractures, 10 distal femoral fractures)	80.5 years (range 70-98)	21 postero-stabilized (9 standard implant and 12 revision endomedullary implants). 5 rotating hinge prostheses.	16.2 months	23% immediate general complications and 15% of local arthroplasty-related complications. The mean active extension deficit was 4.1°. The mean IKS knee score was 82 points. The function score was 54 point. The results referred both to distal femoral and proximal tibial fractures
Malviya *et al.* (9)	2011	25 knees (15 proximal tibial and 10 distal femoral fractures)	80 years (range 67-92)	Depending on surgeon decision.	38.8 months	81% returned to the pre-injury level of activity. 90% of patients were satisfied with the outcome. Mean Knee Society knee score was 90.2; Knee Society function score was 35.5; Oxford Knee score was 39.5; and Short Form (SF)-36 physical function score was 37.3 and mental score 50.6. The results referred both to distal femoral and proximal tibial fractures.
Kini *et al.* (12)	2013	6 lateral tibial plateu fractures + 3 diaphyseal fractures	Not reported	5 postero-stabilized implant, 6 cases of bony defect filled with cement and 2 cases with tantalum metaphyseal cone, all tibial stem (longer in diaphyseal fractures)	26 months	6 patients did not require any walking aid, 2 of them used a stick and one used a walker to ambulate. All 9 patients returned to their preoperative functional level after surgery. Average Range of Movement (ROM) was 114° (95°–125°). Mean Knee Society score was 84. Out of 9 cases 5 were graded as excellent, 3 good and 1 fair

(Table 1) contd.....

Authors	Year	Number of knees	Average age	Type of implants	Mean follow-up	Results
Benazzo *et al.* (8)	2014	2 knees (6 total, 4 distal femoral fractures)	62 years (range 47-76 years)	CCK Zimmer ® and NexGen Zimmer ®	12 months	The mean postoperative clinical KSS was 84 (range 50–100) with 5 patients having good or excellent clinical outcomes. The mean postoperative functional KSS was 78 (range 30–90) with 5 patients having good or excellent results. At the follow-up no x-ray radiolucent lines around the prosthesis were detected. The results referred both to distal femoral and proximal tibial fractures

Conclusion

Complex proximal tibial fractures can be challenging in elderly patients, in whom ORIF can be difficult because of bone quality. Following the same process applied to hip fractures in elderly patients, some authors proposed primary TKA for treating complex proximal tibial fractures in this population, who required early mobilization. The indications are elderly patients with poor bone quality, requiring early mobilization and affected by pre-existing osteoarthritis.

There are few reports on literature describing the results of primary TKAs in this population, with small records and short follow-up. However all the authors agree confirming that this is a safe treatment with good clinical outcomes, but inferior compared to whom obtained in elective TKAs. Really attention has to be due to the indication and the surgeon should expect a higher risk of complications, similar to those reported in revision TKA.

CHRONIC SETTING

Introduction

In almost 50% of cases tibial plateau fractures occur in patients younger than 50 years old [1]. These patients are commonly treated with ORIF, which represents the gold standard. It has been demonstrated that tibial plateau fracture, even if with a good reduction and an apparently perfect "resitutio ad integrum" of the articular surface, increases the risk of early knee osteoarthritis [19, 20]. Wasserstein *et al.* analyzed the incidence of TKAs in their patients, an he observed a 5.3 times higher incidence of knee substitution in patients previously affected by a tibial fracture compared to the normal population (p < 0.0001) in ten years [21]. Rasmussen reported a 21% incidence of arthrosis in the patients treated with ORIF for tibial plateau fractures at a mean of 7.3 years after trauma [22]. The young age of these patients complicates the decision for reconstruction treatment; in patients younger than 60 years old a conservative treatment has to be considered; osteotomies around the knee may decrease pain and slow down the degenerative progression, delaying the time for a total knee arthroplasty [23, 24].

On the contrary, in patients older than 60 years old the replacement should be strongly considered. When approaching a knee replacement in patients with previous surgeries, the strategy should be accurately planned because of different problems: hardware presence, multiple surgical scars, stiffness, bony defects, malalignment, instability, malunions, previous infections and ligaments insufficiency [25]. For those reasons delayed TKA in patients with previous tibial plateau fractures can be challenging, with 26% of and of 21% reoperation rate reported on literature [7].

The indication to TKA should be carefully evaluated for young patients; in literature is widely reported a poor outcome for TKAs implanted in younger than 50 years old [26 - 29].

Preoperative Planning

The planning for a TKA in a post-traumatic arthritis should be the same as in a normal arthroplasty but with some more precaution due to the previous surgery [25]. All variables should be considered and an accurate radiological study has to be performed before surgery. The first step preparing the surgery is a conventional X-Ray in two projections, a sunset view and a weight-bearing long-leg view. In plain radiographs, attention should be paid on bone defects, patellar height, osteolysis, metal hardware position or breakage.

Some authors described the tilt of the tibial plateau in the antero-posterior (AP) and lateral radiographic views as an important technical consideration. Besides the varus-valgus deformity should be assessed, overall in patients affected by malunions, and an osteotomy may be considered before performing arthroplasty in patients with a significant bony deformity above or below the joint line [30]. In our experience it is mandatory to perform a CT scan in order to evaluate the bone quality and the position of the previously implanted hardware. Performing an MRI should be a problem for the low quality of the images due by the interference of the metal hardware. In addition we routinely perform a cultural exam on the synovial fluid in order to exclude infections due to previous surgery.

Surgical Technique

When performing a TKA after a tibial plateau fracture, different problems should be considered: hardware removal, alignment, ligament instabilities and bony defects.

The hardware removal is often necessary because of interference with the implant. The removal can be done either during surgery or before it. Undergoing the removal before the TKA has the inconvenience of exposing the patient to two surgeries; on the other hand the surgeon can be able to take bacteriological samples and carefully evaluate bone quality and stock. Removal of hardware during the TKA has the main advantage to expose the patient to one single surgery, but it can be difficult in cases of voluminous hardware or if a different approach compared to the TKA is needed [31]. The treatment of bony defects should following the same principles discussed in the previous sections.

Osteotomies can be necessary in cases of severe extra-articular deformities. Ligamentous instabilities should be treated when the same principles of elective TKA or revision TKA [17].

Results

There are few reports in literature describing the results of TKA in patients with prior tibial plateau fracture.

Roffi *et al.* in 1990 described their outcomes on 17 cases, with only 8 successful results, concluding that the results may resemble revision rather than primary arthroplasty [30]. Saleh *et al.* reported their results on 15 cases of TKAs implanted at an average of 38.6 months after the fracture. The authors concluded that TKAs after ORIF of a tibial plateau fracture decreases pain and improves knee function, but it is technically demanding and associated to a high failure rate [15].

Weiss *et al.* described the bigger casuistry of TKAs after tibial plateau fracture, concluding that this procedure is affected by higher complication rate and overall poorer outcome when compared with elective TKA [7, 32].

Wu *et al.* reported good clinical outcomes on 15 TKAs with an increased risk of restricted post-operative Range Of Motion (ROM) [33]. Larson *et al.* hypothesized that TKAs performed after infected tibial plateau fractures would have an even higher complication rate if compared with non-infected ones. In their case-control study, with match-paired groups, they concluded that previously infected knees had a 4.1-fol increased risk to require additional procedure [34]. Recently Shearer *et al.* studied the outcomes in 47 knees treated with TKA in post-traumatic arthritis, concluding that the largest improvement in pain and function was detected in patients with isolated intra-articular deformities [35]. Finally Lunebourg *et al.* concluded that patients and surgeons should be aware that clinical outcome and implant survival after TKA for post-traumatic arthritis are lower than after primary elective TKA [36]. (Table **2** shows in summary these results.

Table 2. Literature review describing in detail the results in Total Knee Arthroplasty (TKA) in patients affected by previous tibial plateau fractures.

Authors	Year	Number of knees	Mean follow-up	Results
Roffi *et al.* (39)	1990	17 knees	27 months	8 successful clinical results. 5 major intraoperative or post-operative complications.

(Table 2) contd.....

Authors	Year	Number of knees	Mean follow-up	Results
Saleh *et al.* (15)	2001	15 knees	6.2 years	Average distance from tibial plateau fracture 38.6 months. The average Hospital for Special Surgery knee score was 80 points (range, 44 to 91 points) at the final follow-up. 12 knees were scored as good or excellent.. The average Range of Motion (ROM) was 105 degrees (range, 70 degrees to 135 degrees) compared with 87 degrees (range, 20 degrees to 125 degrees) preoperatively. High infection rate (three patients), patellar tendon disruption (two patients), and postoperative secondary procedures (three patients required closed manipulation).
Weiss *et al.* (7)	2003	62 knees	4.7 years	Main Knee Score of 82.9 and 84 points, respectively. 12 re-operations. 10% of intraoperative and 26% of post-operative complication rate.
Wu *et al.* (33)	2005	15 knees	35 months	The average Knee score was 84 (range, 10-100) and 76 (range, 20-100) points, respectively at the latest follow-up. The mean ROM was94 degree at the latest follow-up. 4 knees required post-operative manipulation under anesthesia. 2 superficial infections.
Shearer *et al.* (35)	2013	47 knees	52 months	Significant improvement in Knee Society Score scores, most of all in pain and functional scores in patients with isolated articular deformities. Soft-tissue defects requiring flap coverage were associated with worsening in the pain score (p= 0.027).
Lunebourg *et al.* (36)	2014	33 knees	11 years	KSS to 77 (SD 15), but the improvement was greater in the control group of elective TKAs (p < 0.001). Postoperative ROM also improved in both groups, from 83° to 108° in the PTA group (p < 0.001) as opposed to 116° to 127° in the PA group (p = 0.001), with lower results in the PTA group (p < 0.001). The survival rate of TKA at 10 years was better in the elective TKAs group (99%, CI: 98-100 vs. 79%, CI: 69-89; p < 0.001).

CONCLUSION

TKAs after tibial plateau fractures are suitable options, with good clinical outcomes reported on literature, but inferior compared to elective TKAs. Alignments, hardware removal, bony defects and ligamentous instabilities are the main problems the surgeons have to consider. There are few reports on literature reporting the results of TKAs after tibial plateau fractures. However most of the authors agree in affirming that is a demanding procedure, with inferior clinical outcomes compared to primary TKAs and associated to higher complication rate.

CONFLICT OF INTEREST

The author confirms that author has no conflict of interest to declare for this publication.

ACKNOWLEDGEMENTS

Declared none.

REFERENCES

[1]   Court-Brown CM, Bugler KE, Clement ND, Duckworth AD, McQueen MM. The epidemiology of open fractures in adults. A 15-year review. Injury 2012; 43(6): 891-7.
[http://dx.doi.org/10.1016/j.injury.2011.12.007] [PMID: 22204774]

[2]   Krupp RJ, Malkani AL, Roberts CS, Seligson D, Crawford CH III, Smith L. Treatment of bicondylar tibia plateau fractures using locked plating *versus* external fixation. Orthopedics 2009; 32(8): orthosupersite.com/view.asp?rID=41916. http://www.ncbi.nlm.nih.gov/pubmed/19708633
[http://dx.doi.org/10.3928/01477447-20090624-11] [PMID: 19708633]

[3]   Bohm ER, Tufescu TV, Marsh JP. The operative management of osteoporotic fractures of the knee: to fix or replace? J Bone Joint Surg Br 2012; 94(9): 1160-9.
[http://dx.doi.org/10.1302/0301-620X.94B9.28130] [PMID: 22933485]

[4]   Honkonen SE. Indications for surgical treatment of tibial condyle fractures. Clin Orthop Relat Res 1994; (302): 199-205.
[PMID: 8168301]

[5]   Scharf S, Christophidis N. Fractures of the tibial plateau in the elderly as a cause of immobility. Aust N Z J Med 1994; 24(6): 725-6.
[http://dx.doi.org/10.1111/j.1445-5994.1994.tb01792.x] [PMID: 7717928]

[6]   Ali AM, El-Shafie M, Willett KM. Failure of fixation of tibial plateau fractures. J Orthop Trauma 2002; 16(5): 323-9.
[http://dx.doi.org/10.1097/00005131-200205000-00006] [PMID: 11972075]

[7]   Weiss NG, Parvizi J, Trousdale RT, Bryce RD, Lewallen DG. Total knee arthroplasty in patients with a prior fracture of the tibial plateau. J Bone Joint Surg Am 2003; 85-A(2): 218-21.
[PMID: 12571297]

[8]   Benazzo F, Rossi SM, Ghiara M, Zanardi A, Perticarini L, Combi A. Total knee replacement in acute and chronic traumatic events. Injury 2014; 45 (Suppl. 6): S98-S104.
[http://dx.doi.org/10.1016/j.injury.2014.10.031] [PMID: 25457327]

[9]   Malviya A, Reed MR, Partington PF. Acute primary total knee arthroplasty for peri-articular knee fractures in patients over 65 years of age. Injury 2011; 42(11): 1368-71.
[http://dx.doi.org/10.1016/j.injury.2011.06.198] [PMID: 21763651]

[10]   Vermeire J, Scheerlinck T. Early primary total knee replacement for complex proximal tibia fractures in elderly and osteoarthritic patients. Acta Orthop Belg 2010; 76(6): 785-93.

[PMID: 21302577]

[11]   Parratte S, Bonnevialle P, Pietu G, Saragaglia D, Cherrier B, Lafosse JM. Primary total knee arthroplasty in the management of epiphyseal fracture around the knee. Orthop Traumatol Surg Res 2011; 97(6) (Suppl.): S87-94.
[http://dx.doi.org/10.1016/j.otsr.2011.06.008] [PMID: 21802385]

[12]   Kini SG, Sathappan SS. Role of navigated total knee arthroplasty for acute tibial fractures in the elderly. Arch Orthop Trauma Surg 2013; 133(8): 1149-54.
[http://dx.doi.org/10.1007/s00402-013-1792-8] [PMID: 23771128]

[13]   Nau T, Pflegerl E, Erhart J, Vecsei V. Primary total knee arthroplasty for periarticular fractures. J Arthroplasty 2003; 18(8): 968-71.
[http://dx.doi.org/10.1016/S0883-5403(03)00280-8] [PMID: 14658099]

[14]   Ries MD. Primary arthroplasty for management of osteoporotic fractures about the knee. Curr Osteoporos Rep 2012; 10(4): 322-7.
[http://dx.doi.org/10.1007/s11914-012-0122-3] [PMID: 23054958]

[15]   Saleh KJ, Sherman P, Katkin P, *et al.* Total knee arthroplasty after open reduction and internal fixation of fractures of the tibial plateau: a minimum five-year follow-up study. J Bone Joint Surg Am 2001; 83-A(8): 1144-8.
[PMID: 11507121]

[16]   Brunner A, Horisberger M, Ulmar B, Hoffmann A, Babst R. Classification systems for tibial plateau fractures; does computed tomography scanning improve their reliability? Injury 2010; 41(2): 173-8.
[http://dx.doi.org/10.1016/j.injury.2009.08.016] [PMID: 19744652]

[17]   Vince KG. Three-Step Technique for Revision Total Knee Arthroplasty. Knee Arthroplasty Handbook 2006; pp. 15-104.Springer New York
[http://dx.doi.org/10.1007/0-387-33531-5_8]

[18]   Nourissat G, Hoffman E, Hemon C, Rillardon L, Guigui P, Sautet A. Total knee arthroplasty for recent severe fracture of the proximal tibial epiphysis in the elderly subject. Rev Chir Orthop Repar Appar Mot 2006; 92(3): 242-7.
[http://dx.doi.org/10.1016/S0035-1040(06)75731-2]

[19]   Honkonen SE. Degenerative arthritis after tibial plateau fractures. J Orthop Trauma 1995; 9(4): 273-7.
[http://dx.doi.org/10.1097/00005131-199509040-00001] [PMID: 7562147]

[20]   Giannoudis PV, Tzioupis C, Papathanassopoulos A, Obakponovwe O, Roberts C. Articular step-off and risk of post-traumatic osteoarthritis. Evidence today. Injury 2010; 41(10): 986-95.
[http://dx.doi.org/10.1016/j.injury.2010.08.003] [PMID: 20728882]

[21]   Wasserstein D, Henry P, Paterson JM, Kreder HJ, Jenkinson R. Risk of total knee arthroplasty after operatively treated tibial plateau fracture: a matched-population-based cohort study. J Bone Joint Surg Am 2014; 96(2): 144-50.
[http://dx.doi.org/10.2106/JBJS.L.01691] [PMID: 24430414]

[22]   Rasmussen PS. Tibial condylar fractures as a cause of degenerative arthritis. Acta Orthop Scand 1972; 43(6): 566-75.
[http://dx.doi.org/10.3109/17453677208991279] [PMID: 4651936]

[23]   Dettoni F, Bonasia DE, Castoldi F, Bruzzone M, Blonna D, Rossi R. High tibial osteotomy *versus* unicompartmental knee arthroplasty for medial compartment arthrosis of the knee: a review of the literature. Iowa Orthop J 2010; 30: 131-40.
[PMID: 21045985]

[24]   Amendola A, Bonasia DE. Results of high tibial osteotomy: review of the literature. Int Orthop 2010; 34(2): 155-60.
[http://dx.doi.org/10.1007/s00264-009-0889-8] [PMID: 19838706]

[25]   Bedi A, Haidukewych GJ. Management of the posttraumatic arthritic knee. J Am Acad Orthop Surg 2009; 17(2): 88-101.
[PMID: 19202122]

[26]   Harrysson OL, Robertsson O, Nayfeh JF. Higher cumulative revision rate of knee arthroplasties in younger patients with osteoarthritis. Clin Orthop Relat Res 2004; (421): 162-8.
[http://dx.doi.org/10.1097/01.blo.0000127115.05754.ce] [PMID: 15123942]

[27]   Gioe TJ, Novak C, Sinner P, Ma W, Mehle S. Knee arthroplasty in the young patient: survival in a community registry. Clin Orthop Relat Res 2007; 464(464): 83-7.
[PMID: 17589362]

[28]   Vince KG. You can do arthroplasty in a young patient, but...: Commentary on articles by John P. Meehan, MD, *et al.*: "Younger age is associated with a higher risk of early periprosthetic joint infection and aseptic mechanical failure after total knee arthroplasty," and Vinay K. Aggarwal, *et al.*: "Revision total knee arthroplasty in the young patient: is there trouble on the horizon?". J Bone Joint Surg Am 2014; 96(7): e58.
[http://dx.doi.org/10.2106/JBJS.M.01596] [PMID: 24695935]

[29]   Meehan JP, Danielsen B, Kim SH, Jamali AA, White RH. Younger age is associated with a higher risk of early periprosthetic joint infection and aseptic mechanical failure after total knee arthroplasty. J Bone Joint Surg Am 2014; 96(7): 529-35.
[http://dx.doi.org/10.2106/JBJS.M.00545] [PMID: 24695918]

[30]   Roffi RP, Merritt PO. Total knee replacement after fractures about the knee. Orthop Rev 1990; 19(7): 614-20.
[PMID: 2381735]

[31]   Windsor RE, Insall JN, Vince KG. Technical considerations of total knee arthroplasty after proximal tibial osteotomy. J Bone Joint Surg Am 1988; 70(4): 547-55.
[PMID: 3356722]

[32]   Weiss NG, Parvizi J, Hanssen AD, Trousdale RT, Lewallen DG. Total knee arthroplasty in post-traumatic arthrosis of the knee. J Arthroplasty 2003; 18(3) (Suppl. 1): 23-6.
[http://dx.doi.org/10.1054/arth.2003.50068] [PMID: 12730923]

[33]   Wu LD, Xiong Y, Yan SG, Yang QS. Total knee replacement for posttraumatic degenerative arthritis of the knee Chinese journal of traumatology = Zhonghua chuang shang za zhi/Chinese Medical Association 2005; 8(4): 1-195.

[34]   Larson AN, Hanssen AD, Cass JR. Does prior infection alter the outcome of TKA after tibial plateau fracture? Clin Orthop Relat Res 2009; 467(7): 1793-9.

[http://dx.doi.org/10.1007/s11999-008-0615-7] [PMID: 19002742]

[35] Shearer DW, Chow V, Bozic KJ, Liu J, Ries MD. The predictors of outcome in total knee arthroplasty for post-traumatic arthritis. Knee 2013; 20(6): 432-6.
[http://dx.doi.org/10.1016/j.knee.2012.12.010] [PMID: 23313556]

[36] Lunebourg A, Parratte S, Gay A, Ollivier M, Garcia-Parra K, Argenson JN. Lower function, quality of life, and survival rate after total knee arthroplasty for posttraumatic arthritis than for primary arthritis. Acta Orthop 2014; 86(2): 94-189.
[PMID: 25350612]

CHAPTER 11

Rehabilitation After Tibial Plateau Fractures

Irene Carnino[1], Annamaria Federico[1], Cecilia Gaido[1], Alessandro Bistolfi[*, 2], and Giuseppe Massazza[1,2]

[1] *School of Rehabilitative Medicine, University of the Studies of Turin. Turin, Italy*

[2] *Hospital Città della Salute e della Scienza , Department of Orthopaedics Traumatology and Rehabilitation, CTO Trauma Centre. Turin, Italy*

Abstract: Tibial plateau fractures are common and severe joint lesions which usually require surgical fixation. They may cause severe postoperative pain and require long hospitalization to provide effective analgesia and to start an appropriate rehabilitation. Specific programs of post-operative rehabilitation are necessary for acceptable recover. Nowadays, well established specific rehabilitation protocols do not exist and treatment is often experience-based. This chapter focuses on physical therapy and on the rehabilitation techniques after tibial plateau fractures; also, it evaluates the effectiveness of the most common techniques.

Keywords: Physical therapies, Physiotherapy, Recover, Rehabilitation, Tibial fracture.

INTRODUCTION

The tibial plateau fracture may take up till 4 months for complete consolidation and it may require up to 6 months or, sometimes, more time to return to the same pre-clinical activity level. This aspect becomes more important when considering that this kind of fracture often happens to socially and working active persons [1]. As described in the previous chapters, fractures of the tibial plateau range from simple undisplaced fractures to complex articular lesions.

---

[*] **Correspondence author Alessandro Bistolfi:** Orthopaedic Surgeon, Hospital Città della Scienza e della Salute, Department of Orthopaedics Traumatology and Rehabilitation, CTO Trauma Centre, Turin, Italy; Tel: +39.011.69331; Email: abistolfi@cittadellasalute.to.it.

Francesco Atzori and Luigi Sabatini (Eds)

The choice of the kind of treatment is a subject for trauma surgeons and obviously it affects the clinical outcome as well as the rehabilitation program. However, the aims of rehabilitation are the same either after conservative and surgical approach, with only a few of specificities: to recover as quickly and as completely as possible the daily activities and, when required, the sport ones.

Since persons with tibial plateau fractures belong to various age brackets with very different demanding (the need of a quick walk for the elderlies and of starting again competitions for the professional sportive patients, respectively) the rehabilitative treatment must be case-specific, based on the characteristics of the patient and on the kind of orthopedic treatment. All these facts underline the importance of the specialist in the rehabilitation for the treatment of a fractured knee: he must consider globally the patients, their clinical situation, co-morbidities, the surgical results and, last but not least, the patient's expectations and goals. Along with the work of the physiotherapist, continued medical surveillance is necessary to evaluate the needs and the progresses of the patient and also to detect as soon as possible any complications.

The rehabilitation program should begin immediately after surgery or after conservative treatment [2] with the following objectives: 1) to control edema and pain, 2) to maintain a correct muscular strength on both legs, 3) to maintain the range of movement of hip and ankle. However, weight bearing and mobilization of the knee are the two key points in the whole rehabilitative process. Since these items are definitely established by the surgeons, an effective and continue collaboration between the medical specialists is greatly recommended to set the timing and the goals of the specific work on the injured knee.

Knee mobilization must be started as early as possible: usually it is authorized by the surgeon, according to the stability of the fracture and the bone quality. When a knee can be mobilized, the Rehabilitation specialist will establish a specific program with the following goals:

1. Progressive recovery of:
    a) range of movement of the knee,
    b) proprioception,

c) muscular strength;
2. Partial and progressive weight bearing on the affected side (usually after 2-3 months according to orthopaedic indications)
3. Recovery of the correct walking pattern (initially with crutches)
4. Recovery of the maximum grade of autonomy in the ADL;
5. Possible return to the previous sport activity.

The immediate identification and treatment of possible serious complications is mandatory (see Red Flags)

It must be considered, that the majority of persons with severe tibial plateau fractures could not come back to their previous level of activity. So patients' awareness is mandatory, specially for the ones playing competitive sports, as this injury could represent a career ender [3]. Overall, a post-injury shift toward activities with less impact has been reported for the majority of people.

Red Flags

- *Non controlled pain*
- *Contention intolerance*
- *Deep-Vein thrombosis*
- *Compartment Syndrome*
- *Infections*
- *Peripheral neurological deficits*

REHABILITATION APPROACH AFTER SURGICAL TREATMENT

Rehabilitation approach can be divided in 3 steps with different goals and programs:

1. Post operative phase: control of pain, reduction of edema, mobilization of other joints.
2. Rehabilitation before the concession of weight bearing: passive and assistive – active mobilization of the injured knee, increasing gradually the range of movement [4], exercises to recover/maintain muscular tono-tropism, treatment of the surgical scar and fibrous adhesions. Walking with crutches.
3. Rehabilitation after the concession of weight bearing: progressive restart of

physiologic walking (at the beginning, loading must be protected by two crutches, then by one and finally without aids) and the recover of a correct step pattern. If possible it will be important the work to recover the correct sportive gesture.

As mentioned, the correct timing of treatment has to be confirmed by the surgeons on the basis of the kind of fracture, surgical intervention and bone quality. Approximately, 10 – 20 days will be necessary to begin the knee mobilization and the recovery of the range of movement and about 3 months for the concession of the weight bearing. In few cases, when a total knee arthroplasty is necessary [5], rehabilitation goals will consist in the praecox recover of the range of movement and loading [6].

However, a great variability in protocols is present in the clinical practice: among a great variety of rehabilitative instruments routinely used in medicine, only a few proved effectiveness. For example, magnetic fields have not demonstrated to be more effective than standard rehabilitation, while hydrokinetic-therapy has been effective in only one clinical trial (6 months follow up in elderly people) [7]. Continuous passive motion has shown good results for the knee range of movement, pain, post operative edema and the lasting of hospitalization at short term [8]. Also cryotherapy, especially when associated to local compression, shows some early benefit but long term positive effect on patients' outcome is still under investigated [9].

REHABILITATION AFTER CONSERVATIVE TREATMENT

In this case the person has to keep a plastered valve or a leg brace, possibly a jointed one, for a variable time from 2 to 4 months after fracture (see chapter 4). During this period, till the removal of the contention, the rehabilitative targets are the control of pain, distal edema and the maintenance of the ankle's range of movement and muscular tropism. Usually, after one month, the mobilization of the knee starts. Obviously, a training to adopt a correct posture, to execute postural passages and to use aids, such as crutches to walk till the concession of weight bearing, will be necessary.

REHABILITATION STRATEGIES

Till the knee mobilization is not permitted by the Orthopaedist, the rehabilitation work begins with passive and active – assistive distal - proximal mobilization by foot fingers to ankle, to preserve a correct range of movement. Table-1 reports the most commonly used physical therapies and summarizes the advantages and contraindications.

Table 1. Physical Therapy.

Physical Therapy	Action and Indications	Contraindications
Cryotherapy	Reduction of edema, haematoma and bleeding Anti-inflammatory action and indirect analgesic one Treatment of muscular spasms and contractures It can be used just before and after physiotherapy sessions to reduce or control pain and possible contractures.	Sensitivity disorders Skin lesions Arterial diseases
Magneto therapy [10]	Analgesic action Reduction of edema Delay of bone consolidation Osteoporosis / pseudo – arthritis	Pace maker Tumors
Tens	Analgesic action (gate control therapy)	wounds Pace maker Metal devices for synthesis
Electrical Stimulation	Muscular ipotonothrophy	Pace maker Tumors Muscular lesions Metal devices for synthesis Skin Lesions Epilepsy

Edema

Moreover, it is essential the control of distal edema, through maintaining the limb elevated (ankle higher than knee, knee higher than hip) and performing the vascular gymnastic exercises that take advantage of the muscular pump to make the venous return easier (Buerger and Hallen exercises). These ones consist in a slow alternated foot dorsiflexion and plantar-flexion keeping for some seconds the maximum range of movement possible; they should be executed in series of 10 repetitions more times per day on the basis of the patients' tolerance. The plantar stimulus is essential to reduce edema: till the weight bearing permission, it can be obtained through wall-side exercises that assure a proprioceptive stimulus. In case of mixed edema (with a lymphatic component) manual lymphatic drainage or vascular bandages can be used. Now, the application of neuromuscular taping is known to be effective as a draining instrument.

Muscular Strength

The patients' education to execute isometric co-contraction of flexors and extensor knee muscles is important to recover muscular tropism [11]. It protects the joint stability avoiding excessive strain and micro-traumas potentially dangerous in an initial phase. When the range of movement has been recovered, the isometric contractions exercises will be carried out at different grades of range of movement, training muscles at different muscular lengths.

In a second time, isotonic contractions will be requested. At the beginning they will be concentric and in closed kinetic chain, then they will be eccentric ones. If a marked weakness is present, electrical stimulation can avoid a major muscular mass loss. It's useful to practice these exercises bilaterally, to make learning and memorization of movement easier and to maintain a correct muscular strength and tropism.

Range of movement

Following the individualized timing steps given by the Orthopaedic specialist, in every single case the leg brace will be unblocked, or the valve removed, to begin the recovery of knee range of movement. An initial passive mobilization will be followed by an active – assisted one, always in absence of pain. During treatment it's important to obtain the person's attention and compliance, avoiding muscular spasms and contractures that could obstruct the physiological recovery. Patients have to be educated to an active cooperation with therapists, through the home training of the learned exercises.

Red Flag: Post Traumatic Stiffness

The stiffness of a knee is the result of a combination of factors: soft tissue contracture, fracture location and extra bone formation.

Major complications may be rare but it has been reported that 20% of the patients undergoing total knee replacement [12] had knee stiffness at twelve months. In many studies a strong relationship between the recovery range of motion and the functional outcomes after both elective and emergency surgery is demonstrated. Multiple risk factors of stiff knee after total knee replacement are known [13, 14] but there are not enough studies about predictive factors after the treatment of tibial fractures. The risk factors for knee stiffness are the lesion of the extensor muscles, fasciotomy, incomplete wound care, and the execution of three or more surgical procedures on the limb. Multiple other factors such as age, sex, side of injury, mechanism of injury, length of intensive care unit stay, associated head injury, rehabilitation technique (*e.g.* use of continuous passive motion), and discharge home versus to a rehabilitation facility found to have no impact on the outcome [15] . Post traumatic stiffness must be avoided and prevented with all means.

Walk Ability

To permit a correct orthostatic position and walking recovery, it is mandatory to support the anti-gravity and hip establishing muscles (gluteus, abductors, and quadriceps) because, without them, it is impossible to achieve a correct step scheme. After the loading permission, rehabilitation in orthostatic position will begin, initially with a double support. To make the person aware about the load distribution on the two limbs, balances can be used. In a second time they can be useful for loading transfer exercises, preparatory to the different step phases.

The proposal of using joint proprioceptive exercises, through the use of instable plans and computerized platforms, is mandatory for a good rehabilitative result. A good proprioceptive recovery can insure good knee stability.

Hydrokinesitherapy

Hydrokinesitherapy, after the surgical wound healing, can be introduced in different rehabilitative moments. Indeed water properties, at a therapeutic temperature (about 35°), can be used to: a) reduce joint pain and, if possible, muscular stiffness; b) make the tissue sliding easier; c) increase muscular strengthening; d) work with less pain e) make the recovery of walking and orthostatic position exercises faster (with reduced load).

PHARMACOLOGICAL THERAPY

Pain Control

A good pain control is basic to safeguard patients' compliance to rehabilitative treatment. During the post operative period it has been demonstrated that the use of COX2 inhibitors permits a best pain control with a faster knee flexion recovery, a reduction of hospitalization time and a less numerous assumptions of narcotic drugs. Moreover, during the all rehabilitation time and the coming back home, a good antalgic therapy must be assured to the patients. When the inflammatory component is prevalent, anti-inflammatory drugs can be used, while if the painful component is prevalent, specific antalgic drugs (also morphine-derivates), chosen on the basis of the NRS scale and the pain pyramid, can be used (OMS) [13].

Prophylaxis for Thrombosis and Osteoporosis

Deep venous thrombosis (DVT) is a serious potential complication following major orthopaedic surgery. Many different forms of therapy have been proposed and optimal strategies include pharmacologic and mechanical approaches such as graduated compression stockings and intermittent pneumatic compression [14]. Timing and duration of the application of prophylactic agents has also been determined to have a significant effect to prevent the development of DVT. Early prophylaxis in surgical patients has been associated with significant reductions in postoperative venous thrombosis. Initiation of therapy within 8 hours after surgery has the greatest effect and is recommended by the American College of Chest Physicians (ACCP). Extended out-of-hospital prophylaxis for until full weight bearing is recommended to decrease venous thrombosis rates without major bleeding issues. Traditional anticoagulant drugs such as low-molecular-weight-heparin (LMWH) and warfarin are indicated to stop the coagulation process to prevent a thrombosis. Finally it is important to underline that new generation drugs can target a single coagulation's agent.

Supplementation with Calcium and Vitamin D, to make the bone consolidation easier, can be indicated. Vitamin D, through its action on calcium metabolism, is essential for bone physiology [15]. Vitamin D is important to reach a good functional outcome and to reduce the risks of new fractures. However we must remember that is very important remove specific risk factors (like hypocalcaemia, smoke, sedentary life) to prevent osteoporosis. The drugs for the treatment of osteoporosis should be used only when the benefits overcome the risks. Vitamin D and calcium supplementation, a correct nutrition, physical exercise, and also a treatment against osteoporosis, can ensure the optimal recovery and survival [16].

Viscosupplementation

The tibial plateau fracture can lead to knee osteoarthritis: appropriate management decisions for minimizing pain and improving physical function are important. Hyaluronic acids knee injections have become a common tool for the management of OA of the knee but a lot of studies demonstrate quite low effects on the regeneration of the cartilage and on the pain relief [17]. On the contrary, serious adverse events have been correlated to the injections of Hyaluronic acids [18]. Although still questionable and under debate, the hypothesis to support the cartilage with chondro-derivates must be considered.

Moreover, in case of major risks of consolidation delay and possible development of Complex Regional Pain Syndrome (CRPS) [19, 20] pharmacological and rehabilitative therapies can be used. Pharmacological approach can include anti-inflammatory drugs, bisphosphonates and Calcitonin to reduce pain. Rehabilitative multi-professional approach consists of physiotherapy with active assisted exercises avoiding pain and muscular fatigue development, physical therapy. It's possible to draw upon sympathetic blocks with local anesthetics and botulinum toxin A.

DISCUSSION AND CONCLUSION

There are specific patients' and fractures' factors that influence the final recovery result: trauma intensity, fracture morphology, bone quality, the associated capsule-ligament injuries, age, comorbidities and clinical conditions of the patients: these factors appear to be able to affect prognosis, independently from the type of treatment undertaken. However, it must be remembered that the functional outcome is essentially due to the quality of fracture's anatomical reduction, joint stability obtained and the correct recovery of the axes. Failure or incomplete achievement of these objectives may facilitate a progression to osteoarthritis. Furthermore, it must be considered that in approximately 50% of cases the tibial plateau fracture resulting from high-energy trauma correlates to ligament, meniscal and capsular injuries, which are generally treated in a second surgical time, limiting the results obtained in a first stage rehabilitation.

The recovery time and the choice of the rehabilitation program may be affected, even considerably, by the onset of early and late complications. Among the early complications the most common are compartmental syndrome, vascular lesions, delayed wound healing, infections, deep venous thrombosis and peripheral nerve deficits. All these cases require ortho-trauma surgical management and may delay the beginning of the rehabilitation. The most important late complications are knee instability, angular deformities, consolidation disorders, pseudo-arthrosis, osteoarthritis and knee stiffness. While the first four instances are subjects for the orthopaedic intervention again, the last two ones show different paths : osteoarthritis often is an unavoidable consequence derived from the damage of the cartilage. So, the patient must be informed and forewarned. On the other side, stiffness is a complication that must be fought with all means. Timing is a key point: when the rigidity is structured and adherences established, only a few persons can carry out the physical therapy. On the contrary, early mobilization, along with adequate pain control through all methods (pharmacological and physical therapies) is usually effective in maintaining or recovering an acceptable to excellent range of movement.

CONFLICT OF INTEREST

The author confirms that author has no conflict of interest to declare for this publication.

ACKNOWLEDGEMENTS

Declared none.

REFERENCES

[1]   Albuquerque RP, Hara R, Prado J, Schiavo L, Giordano V, do Amaral NP. Epidemiological study on

tibial plateau fractures at a level I trauma center. Acta Ortop Bras 2013; 21(2): 109-15.
[http://dx.doi.org/10.1590/S1413-78522013000200008] [PMID: 24453653]

[2]   Gausewitz S, Hohl M. The significance of early motion in the treatment of tibial plateau fractures. Clin Orthop Relat Res 1986; (202): 135-8.
[PMID: 3955941]

[3]   Kraus TM, Martetschläger F, Müller D, *et al.* Return to sports activity after tibial plateau fractures: 89 cases with minimum 24-month follow-up. Am J Sports Med 2012; 40(12): 2845-52.
[http://dx.doi.org/10.1177/0363546512462564] [PMID: 23118120]

[4]   Hill AD, Palmer MJ, Tanner SL, Snider RG, Broderick JS, Jeray KJ. Use of continuous passive motion in the postoperative treatment of intra-articular knee fractures. J Bone Joint Surg Am 2014-16; 96(14): e118.
[http://dx.doi.org/10.2106/JBJS.M.00534] [PMID: 25031380]

[5]   Bohm ER, Tufescu TV, Marsh JP. The operative management of osteoporotic fractures of the knee: to fix or replace? J Bone Joint Surg Br 2012; 94(9): 1160-9.
[http://dx.doi.org/10.1302/0301-620X.94B9.28130] [PMID: 22933485]

[6]   Civinini R, Carulli C, Matassi F, Villano M, Innocenti M. Total knee arthroplasty after complex tibial plateau fractures. Chir Organi Mov 2009; 93(3): 143-7.
[PMID: 19711154]

[7]   Giaquinto S, Ciotola E, Dall'Armi V, Margutti F. Hydrotherapy after total knee arthroplasty. A follow-up study. Arch Gerontol Geriatr 2010; 51(1): 59-63.
[http://dx.doi.org/10.1016/j.archger.2009.07.007] [PMID: 19735951]

[8]   Alkire MR, Swank ML. Use of Inpatient continuous passive motion versus no CPM in computer assisted total knee artroplasty. Orthop Nurs 2010; 29: 1.
[http://dx.doi.org/10.1097/NOR.0b013e3181c8ce23] [PMID: 20142683]

[9]   Adie S, Naylor JM, Harris IA. Cryotherapy after total knee arthroplasty. A systematic review and meta Analysis of randomized controlled trials. The Journal of Arthroplasty 2010; 25(5): 709-15.

[10]   Błaszczak E, Franek A, Taradaj J, Widuchowski J, Klimczak J. Assessment of the efficacy and safety of low frequency, low intensity magnetic fields in patients after knee endoprosthesis plasty. Part 1: in vitro safety. Bioelectromagnetics 2009; 30(2): 159-62.
[http://dx.doi.org/10.1002/bem.20457] [PMID: 19009533]

[11]   Boccardi S, Lissoni A. Cinesiologia. Roma: Società Editrice Universo 1984.

[12]   Fischer HB, Simanski CJ, Sharp C, *et al.* PROSPECT Working Group. A procedure-specific systematic review and consensus recommendations for postoperative analgesia following total knee arthroplasty. Anaesthesia 2008; 63(10): 1105-23.
[http://dx.doi.org/10.1111/j.1365-2044.2008.05565.x] [PMID: 18627367]

[13]   Relief CP. "With a guide to opioid availability". Geneva: WHO 1996.

[14]   Falck-Ytter Y, Francis CW, Johanson NA, *et al.* American College of Chest Physicians. Prevention of VTE in orthopedic surgery patients: Antithrombotic therapy and prevention of thrombosis, American college of chest physicians evidence-based clinical practice guidelines. Chest 9. 2012; 141 (2): e278S-325S.

[15]   Handoll H. Update of a systematic review of vitamin D for preventing osteoporotic fractures. Inj Prev 2009; 15(3): 213-7.
[http://dx.doi.org/10.1136/ip.2009.021576] [PMID: 19494105]

[16]   Iolascon G, Di Pietro G, Gimigliano F. Vitamin D supplementation in fractured patient: how, when and why. Clin Cases Miner Bone Metab 2009; 6(2): 120-4.
[PMID: 22461160]

[17]   Divine JG, Zazulak BT, Hewett TE. Viscosupplementation for knee osteoarthritis: a systematic review. Clin Orthop Relat Res 2007; 455(455): 113-22.
[http://dx.doi.org/10.1097/BLO.0b013e31802f5421] [PMID: 17159579]

[18]   Rutjes AW, Jüni P, da Costa BR, Trelle S, Nüesch E, Reichenbach S. Viscosupplementation for osteoarthritis of the knee: a systematic review and meta-analysis. Inglese (U.S.A.) Ann Intern Med 2012; 157(3): 180-91.
[http://dx.doi.org/10.7326/0003-4819-157-3-201208070-00473]

[19]   O'Connell NE, Wand BM, McAuley J, Marston L, Moseley GL. Interventions for treating pain and disability in adults with complex regional pain syndrome. Cochrane Database Syst Rev 2013; 4: CD009416.
[PMID: 23633371]

[20]   Varenna M, Adami S, Sinigaglia L. Bisphosphonates in complex regional pain syndrome type i: how do they work? Inglese (U.S.A.) Clin Exp Rheumatol 2014; 32(4): 451-4.
[PMID: 24959990]

[21]   Timmers TK, van der Ven DJ, de Vries LS, van Olden GD. Functional outcome after tibial plateau fracture osteosynthesis: a mean follow-up of 6 years. Knee 2014; 21(6): 1210-5.
[http://dx.doi.org/10.1016/j.knee.2014.09.011] [PMID: 25311514]

Appendix

ACCP	=	American College of Chest Physicians
ACL	=	Anterior Cruciate Ligament
ADL	=	Activity Daily Life
AO	=	Arbeitsgemeinschaft für Osteosynthesefragen (Association for the Study of Internal Fixation)
AP	=	Antero-Posterior
ARIF	=	Arthroscopic Reduction Internal Fixation
ASA	=	American Society of Anaesthesiologists
CRPS	=	Complex Regional Pain Syndrome
CT	=	Computerized Tomography
DCO	=	Damage Control Orthopaedics
DVT	=	Deep Venous Thrombosis
G-A	=	Gustilo-Anderson
IKDC	=	International Knee Documentation Committee
IKS	=	International Knee Society Rating System
K-WIRES	=	Kirschner Wires
LCL	=	Lateral Collateral Ligament
MCL	=	Medial Collateral Ligament
MDCT	=	Multiple Detector Computed Tomography
MRI	=	Magnetic Resonance Imaging
OA	=	Osteoarthritis
OTA	=	Orthopaedic Trauma Association
ORIF	=	Open Reduction Internal Fixation
PCL	=	Posterior Cruciate Ligament
ROM	=	Range of Movement
TA	=	Tibialis Anterior Muscle
TKA	=	Total Knee Arthroplasty
TKR	=	Total Knee Replacement

SUBJECT INDEX

A

AO classification 15, 18, 19

Approach 27, 30, 38, 55, 56, 59, 79, 90, 106, 109, 113, 115, 123, 129, 130, 147, 148, 171, 178, 179, 185

Arthritis 16, 47, 49, 55, 60, 106, 118, 123, 143, 157, 165, 170, 171, 181

Arthroplasty i, 43, 100, 155, 159, 160, 162, 180, 187, 189

Articular fracture 3, 4, 7, 43, 65

B

Balloon i, iii, 77, 79, 80, 83, 89

Bony avulsion 66, 131, 132, 149, 152, 153

C

Cartilage 16, 17, 35, 40, 42, 43, 57, 68, 69, 72, 77, 79, 83, 86, 87, 185, 186

Cast 27, 40, 43, 44, 56, 57, 59, 60, 106, 112

Compartment syndrome 3, 6, 20, 21, 23, 43, 68, 72, 73, 92, 98, 105, 108, 134, 139, 179

Computer tomography 24, 161

Conservative i, iii, 56, 147, 149, 169, 178, 180

D

Damage control i, 103, 106, 127, 128, 189

Diagnosis i, iii, iv, 24, 25, 27, 30, 35, 39, 46, 58, 61, 78, 110, 113, 131, 134, 138, 139, 141, 143, 144, 157

E

Elderly 4, 9, 13, 18, 19, 24, 25, 46, 60, 61, 78, 79, 82, 83, 86, 88, 97, 114, 117, 165, 168, 173, 174, 180

Epidemiology i, iii, iv, 11, 49, 135, 173

External fixation iii, 13, 23, 45, 56, 58, 59, 99, 103, 106, 114, 173

I

Imaging 6, 10, 12, 14, 15, 24, 25, 27, 34, 38, 39, 46, 48, 57, 61, 88, 92, 96, 98, 131, 134, 156, 189

Injuries 27, 30, 32, 35, 55, 56, 59, 61, 64, 73, 74, 93, 96, 97, 99, 100, 103, 105, 108, 111, 113, 115, 149, 151, 152, 185, 186

Internal fixation i, iii, 12, 27, 41, 58, 74, 75, 87, 88, 90, 93, 94, 96, 99, 101, 102, 105, 108, 109, 112, 126, 127, 129, 130, 137, 139, 155, 159, 160, 162, 163, 174, 189

K

Knee arthroscopy i, 65

L

Ligamentous injuries 10, 32, 35, 131, 132, 138, 139, 143, 144, 149, 152

M

Magnetic resonance imaging 6, 10, 12, 24, 30, 34, 39, 48, 61, 96, 140, 156, 189

Management 11, 13, 14, 24, 25, 30, 65, 88, 89, 97, 131, 140, 185-187

Mechanism injury 3

Meniscal tears 5, 66, 73, 131, 132, 135, 137, 141, 158

N

Nonoperative 3, 12, 18, 40, 135, 140, 149, 156

www.ingramcontent.com/pod-product-compliance
Lightning Source LLC
Chambersburg PA
CBHW041700210326
41598CB00007B/481